Body
Architect

A Real-World Guide to Ignite Your Fitness, Look Awesome Naked, Quiet the Inner Voices of Self-Doubt, & Design a Lifestyle on Your Own Terms

By Julian Hayes II

Publishing services provided by:

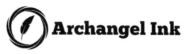

ISBN: 1532781946
ISBN-13: 978-1532781940

Dedication

This is for you, Mom & Dad. Thanks for always being there for me, no matter how complicated and frustrating I can be at times. And for patiently allowing me to find my way.

Medical Disclaimer

The following information is intended for general information and entertainment purposes only. Individuals should always see their health care provider before implementing the suggestions recommended in this book. This book is not intended to replace sound professional medical advice or to treat specific maladies. Any application of the material and recommendations set forth in the following pages is at the reader's discretion and is his or her sole responsibility. The publishers and author assume no liability.

Your Free Gift

As a way of saying thanks for your purchase, I'm offering a free 5-day fat loss course titled *Fail-Proof Fat Loss*.

In *Fail-Proof Fat Loss*, you'll discover the essential techniques that will guarantee success in your fat loss goals without having your daily lifestyle thrown upside down. You will learn how to lose fat using a sustainable and intelligent approach, thus preventing the chances of rebound weight gain. Join the community and kick-start your fat loss with this free 5-day course at theartoffitnessandlife.com

Contents

Section I

Intro: All Hope Isn't Lost; It's Time to Rise Up

Your Current Reality and Why This Book is for You

"The secret to change is to focus all your energy, not on fighting the old, but on building the new."

—Socrates

When was the last time you felt amazing while sporting your healthiest weight, excelling at work, and living a lifestyle you were proud of?

Think about that for a minute.

In today's world, we're busier and more distracted than ever. Balancing your career, relationships, family responsibilities, and social life while attempting to integrate a consistent exercise routine into the mix becomes the latest installment of *Mission Impossible.*

Many of us tell ourselves it's either fitness or our professional careers. We tell ourselves it's fitness or a fulfilling social life. We tell ourselves that once we get our lives together, we'll start exercising.

We tell ourselves that the ability to build a body we can be proud of while living a rich lifestyle designed on our terms is a fairy tale.

That type of mindset and attitude needs to go. Like, seriously, take a couple seconds and flush that thought down the toilet.

In this book, you're going to be presented with a set of realistic and doable options to improve your health and fitness while living a lifestyle on your own terms.

We're going to emphasize the fundamentals of training and nutrition. In addition, we're going to explore the essential mindset and lifestyle principles you'll need to succeed with fitness. Without a big-picture understanding of the fundamentals, succeeding in fitness is a pipe dream.

In this book, you're going to improve physically, but also you're going to improve both mentally and emotionally.

I know what you're thinking. This sounds like I'm blowing smoke up your rear while delivering empty bags of motivation. I get it. There's a lot of fluff and empty promises in the health and fitness space.

You perhaps have some initial questions, concerns, and other preconceived beliefs about fitness—as you should.

Are you perhaps thinking…

"What about my career?" "What about my family and friends who couldn't care less about health & fitness?" "What about eating out with friends and my social life?" "What about nutrition? I don't want to eat or train like a bodybuilder (I get it, I don't want to be the Tupperware king either)." "What about sacrifices? Do I have to let go of all my favorite treats and activities?" "I've struggled with fitness in the past; why should I even try again?"

These are valid questions and without addressing these concerns, you won't be able to become the architect of your own body or life.

The good news about fitness is that there are a multitude of methods that will lead you to success. The biggest problem that people make is losing their identity in the process of integrating fitness into their lives.

This is unnecessary.

At the end of the day, what's the point of making dramatic improvements in your health and fitness if you can't enjoy yourself due to becoming a prisoner to the process?

However, before we move on, just who the heck am I?

Why Should You Listen to Me?

As a student of health, nutrition, and fitness for over ten years, I've learned a plethora of lessons.

Some lessons were physically taxing, some mentally taxing and emotionally depleting—requiring months of recovery in certain instances.

Taking shots of olive oil on a daily basis, eating a dozen eggs every day, completely eliminating carbs (terrible idea), avoiding sugar at all costs (not necessary), emotionally eating everything in sight, being suckered into numerous fad diets—I've conducted my fair share of random dietary experiments.

I've been the perfect little fitness soldier at times, and on the opposite end of the spectrum, I've completely fallen off the fitness wagon.

I've tried bodybuilding routines, full body routines, circuits, and every other possible training regimen you can imagine (except prancercise).

Fitness, at one point in time, was my ruler and I was its servant—willing to do anything and everything to make progress.

Letting fitness rule my life caused me to miss many awesome experiences in college and early adulthood. I missed out on the opportunity to date wonderful women, leading to lonely weekend nights playing video games and watching cheesy romantic comedies (proudly representing for all the hopeless romantics) all in the name of staying within my macros and getting those gains.

However, all wasn't lost. Throughout the journey, I gained valuable insights and real-world knowledge, which has allowed me to prevent others from making these same mistakes along with saving them time (our most precious asset).

I've personally applied and tested each of the strategies in this book throughout the years and the majority of these strategies are implemented with each client I consult and coach.

I Know Something About You Already

Because you've picked up this book, I already have a better understanding of you as a person.

You want to level up in life. You want better health. You want to make fitness a part of your life without chaos ensuing in the other facets of your life as a result. You want to simplify nutrition.

You want to make training efficient and effective. You want a physique that not only performs well, but one you're proud to show off. You want more confidence. You want happiness and peace. You want mental clarity, thus allowing you to create meaningful work to share. You want sustainable, healthy habits. You want to remove the blocks that are holding you back from greatness.

I know there's a fire inside of you that's waiting to be unleashed. I know, and deep down I think you know there is much more to you than what is being currently represented.

What's All This Stuff About My Personal Life in a Fitness Book?

Great question! Personally, I'm interested in multiple disciplines and I'm on a quest to be a Renaissance man. But whatever your situation, health and fitness intersect with every facet of your life.

Health and fitness are the most powerful and essential assets needed to live a rich and fulfilling life. Pretend fitness is the head of an octopus and the tentacles are the other facets of your life. Without the head, the tentacles aren't going to operate.

Fitness is the foundation to doing anything. Achieving a fitness goal creates ripples within your life, increases confidence, and allows you to share your creative superpowers with the world at maximum efficiency and effectiveness.

I started the Art of Fitness and Life for this very reason—we all have a plethora of specific challenges going on within our lives that takes us away from exercising. If we weren't faced with these individual challenges throughout our days, we would all have eye-catching physiques and perfect health biomarkers.

Our toughest challenge isn't completing our sets of squats and deadlifts, but instead it is learning how to incorporate exercise into our lives without throwing everything else out of order.

A Brief Origin Story for This Book

For the majority of 2015, I was at a low point with my fitness, confidence, healthy habits, and general well-being. I lost my fitness identity and needed to pick myself up off the floor.

Though I'd been lifting for over a decade, I lost sight of the essentials. My physical and athletic abilities couldn't save me once I became emotionally and mentally depleted.

I decided to write some letters and essays, which would serve as reminders about what a fit and healthy lifestyle encompasses.

Before I started, I wrote one question on my whiteboard that would serve as the overarching theme: "If I were new to fitness or had lost my way with fitness, how could I get fitness back into my life while being emotionally and mentally healthy and living a good lifestyle"?

Each point in this book represents an essential aspect of establishing a sustainable fitness habit without upending your life or becoming an emotional wreck.

The Goal of This Book

My goal for this book is to release your worries, fears, confusion, and doubts about thriving in fitness while living a fulfilling life.

If you're someone who has fallen on tough times with your fitness, this book will help you start standing on your own feet again.

If you're a total beginner, this book will provide the necessary roadmap to integrating yourself into the world of health and fitness.

My Promise to You

I promise that if you start reading this book on a Wednesday afternoon, by Wednesday night, you'll already be experiencing results (provided you participate in the end-missions).

I promise that if you follow these strategies, you'll become the architect of your own body without sacrificing your entire lifestyle and identity.

How to Use This Book

This book is best suited as a reference guide to remind you of the necessary and essential principles of health and fitness.

My suggestion is to read it from start to finish the first time through. Take note of the strategies that stand out to you and let those serve as your initial focal points.

Afterwards, use this guide to refer back to specific missions (i.e., strategy points) as you continually improve your habits.

It's nearly impossible to make a complete 180 with your daily habits and behaviors. With this in mind, circle a couple of strategies you want to improve on and master those before moving onto another set of strategies.

Here's a warning before we start

Everything sounds great so far. A six-pack, sexy legs, perky glutes, improved health markers, and increased confidence is on the way.

But first, let's put on those brakes for a brief public service announcement.

Fitness isn't easy. It takes a lot of hard work. Living a lifestyle on your own terms while building the body you want requires you to be patient, meticulous, mindful, and intentional with your actions and decisions.

You might be a little uncomfortable at times, and that's okay. That signals growth.

Succeeding in fitness starts with equipping yourself with a proper mindset, taking into account your specific background, assessing your current exercising levels, and then constructing a fitness identity that considers these initial factors.

What you won't find here is a recommendation for fad diets or any type of diet that helps you lose 30lbs in 15 days. This book does not contain any ancient dietary nutritional hacks promising to boost your metabolism by 300% or any other outlandish claims.

You won't be provided with a one-size-fits-all, militant, step-by-step meal plan to follow. You're not a robot nor are you the same as the next reader.

You won't be provided with a secret insider's workout plan promising to whip you into shape in 25 days (there isn't such a thing). You won't be provided Band-Aid solutions delivering you immediate gratification (those will only unravel in the long term).

With that said, at the conclusion of reading this book, you'll emerge with an open mind, a greater sense of adventure, increased confidence about succeeding in fitness, and a desire for constant self-improvement. After reading, you won't blindly follow or believe what you see on the TV, read on the Internet, or hear from your coworkers, gurus, and the random Joes and Janes at the gym.

Most important, you're going to know how to start and sustain a fitness habit while living an optimal lifestyle designed on your own terms. You're going to become the emperor of your own life.

Every day brings about the chance to level up, improve your eating habits, start exercising, go after that dream job, or ask out that dream girl and/or guy you've been eyeing. Time is precious—it's time to stop waiting.

While these opportunities are in front of us each day, it's pivotal that you understand none of these goals will happen if you don't take action and seize the moment. Motivation is cool. Talking about what you want to do is exciting. But taking action is the only way to obtain results.

It's time to rise up, reclaim your life, and build the body you desire. It's time to become the superhero of your own life.

Section II

Mindset

"Whether you think you can or think you can't—you are right."

—Henry Ford

You have the world's sexiest and most elaborate training program. Check.

You have a nutritional program designed for the stars.

Check.

Obtaining your sexy body isn't a matter of what if; it's only a matter of when. Right?

Not exactly.

In fact, you're most likely heading down a one-way street toward disappointment. While this approach may offer amazing tools, the most important aspect to any successful transformation hasn't been mentioned.

Your mindset.

If you aren't prepping your mind for success, then you have a 0% chance of succeeding. Before changing your external world (aka your body), you must change your internal world (aka your mindset).

I understand the word mindset (or more correctly, being mindful) is tossed around more than celebrities switch hook-up partners or the local frat performs keg stands, but your mindset, nevertheless, is your tipping point.

Our mindsets possess the power to guide us toward happiness and success or lead us into the pits of sorrow and frustration, where we ultimately end up stuck in a puddle of mediocrity. Our mindsets are the engine to helping us build the body we want. Just as a car won't go far without a proper working engine, you won't come close to building your desired body without a proper mindset.

A proper mindset is one of growth, where achievements are possible, regardless of the initial circumstances or initial skill levels. As Dr. Carol Dweck, author of *Mindset: The New Psychology of Success* states, "A mindset change isn't about picking up a few pointers here and there. It's about seeing things in a new way."

Changing your mindset is the first of many steps that will pave the way to becoming the architect of your own body.

Even with a proper mindset, your journey won't be full of kittens, sunshine, and rainbows 100% of the time. But going into battle with a positive and optimistic point of view helps you survive those less-than-desirable times and inevitable resistances.

Before moving any further in this book, take a brief moment and pause. Allow your mind to open up and let go of past situations and shortfalls. As Franklin D. Roosevelt states, "The only limits to our realization of tomorrow will be our doubts of today."

Cleanse yourself of any past setbacks and limiting beliefs, and enter your new era with a fresh slate.

It's time to engineer a proper mindset that will guide you to designing a world-class body while being invulnerable to resistances, temptations, and any other obstacle that stands in your way.

Strategy #1: Every Origin Story Starts With a Why

Since the beginning of time, every superhero, famous painter, musician, writer, and great leader who's sought remarkable feats all have one commonality.

What is it?

They have a clear and defined "why."

When I started The Art of Fitness & Life, my mission was clear—to help one million people become the architects of their own bodies and lives, thus allowing fitness and health to serve as their launching pads to making their unique dent in the universe.

When Bruce Wayne becomes Batman, he has a specific mission of protecting Gotham from the criminals of the city.

Peter Parker becomes Spider-Man because of the wisdom that "with great power comes great responsibility", shared by Uncle Ben before his sudden death.

Being equipped with a deeply rooted "why" allows you to stay committed to the process because you have an unending belief in and reasoning for what you're going after.

Before you step foot into the gym, update your gym wardrobe, go grocery shopping, update your status on Facebook declaring your newfound commitment for fitness, or buy a gym membership, you need to get intimate with your "why."

Know your "why" inside and out. Your "why" will inform everything you do.

Why do you want to reach your fitness goals? What will achieving your fitness goals bring to your life? Go beyond surface level with your "why." It's true, losing fifteen pounds might expose your abs to the public or help you look stunning in that bikini by the poolside.

But superficial metrics fade over time and working out for the approval of others is a dangerous game to play. The goal of being the hottest person at the beach or in your city is a losing strategy (here's the thing, there's always going to be someone hotter and leaner—get over it).

Superficial motivators aren't enough to carry you through the long term, especially when life starts to throw random jabs, hooks, and roundhouses at you from various and unsuspected angles.

When first meeting with a client, I challenge them to go beyond surface level and get to the nitty gritty of why they want to succeed with their particular fitness goal.

Use the process outlined below to dig deeper into your motivation for getting started on your new fitness path (of course, everyone's answers will differ). Your goal is to develop a bond with your "why "that's so strong, you'll become one and the same.

1. Question: Why do you want to start working out?

Answer: To look amazing naked, have more sex, impress all my peers, and strangers at the beach.

2. Question: Why do you want to look amazing naked, impress your peers, and various strangers at the beach?

Answer: So I will feel more confident about myself. As well, I want to increase the value I bring to the world.

3. Question: Why do you want to feel more confident about yourself and what you represent to the world?

Answer: So I can have faith that I can accomplish anything I go after.

4. Question: Why do you want to have faith in yourself when it comes to going after anything you try to accomplish?

Answer: So I can live the life that I've visualized over and over in my head—the one where I have a body I'm proud of while excelling in my work.

One of the most important questions you need to ask yourself and be truthful with through this process is, "What am I willing to give up?"

Jim Morrison once said in one of my favorite songs, "The Soft Parade" that "we want the world and we want it now." Unfortunately, fitness doesn't operate under this type of immediate gratification ideology.

To reach your physique goals, sacrifices are a necessity. You might not be able to attend as many happy hours, gorge yourself on slices of cake in the office, or heavily binge drink with your friends at the tailgate.

But that's ok.

Why?

Because your "why" is worth more than just a couple hours of fun that fades away and leaves you with a headache and in desperate search for Advil.

Notice how deep the answers drilled into your "why."

Digging deep into your "why" ensures that when you're having a lazy day, and Chinese takeout and Netflix sounds like the perfect pairing, your trusty "why" will be there to gently tap you on the shoulder and remind you that you're on a mission and to not give in to the dark side of temptations.

Your mission, should you choose to accept

Take some time today and become intimate with your "why." Be 100% clear on why and what you want to accomplish with your fitness goal. There is no right or wrong answer. Paint a picture of what fitness looks like for you, not for anyone else and not what society tries to engineer into your head.

Strategy #2: Marvin Gaye & the Power of Belief & Persistence

"I don't like to follow my footsteps and my shadow. Singers are afraid to branch out and try something new and exciting. But I wasn't."

—Marvin Gaye

Throughout the 1960s, Marvin Gaye was a hit-making machine melting every woman's heart with songs such as "Ain't Nothing Like The Real Thing," "Stubborn Kind of Fellow," "How Sweet It Is," "I Heard It Through The Grapevine," and "You're All I Need To Get By." Along the way, he decided to break the mold.

Gaye felt compelled to dig into his artistry. He wanted to produce himself, instead of having it done by the same people at Motown. Gaye had an idea for an experimental concept album and if the album tanked, it could potentially mark the end to his illustrious career.

Berry Gordy, the head honcho at Motown records, didn't approve of this idea. Motown had a proven formula at that time, which consisted of lightweight and warmhearted records, radio-friendly songs, neat and clean verses, and albums that functioned as a collection of singles.

Despite the risk, the chatter from those at Motown, and the inner voices inside whispering doubt, Gaye remained firm on his idea.

This album was going to be the complete opposite of the Motown formula: socially conscious songs that discussed the Vietnam War, social oppression and injustice, drug abuse, inner-city violence, and unemployment. Ultimately, it would make America look at itself in the mirror.

This album wasn't going to be radio friendly. It was going to be a cohesive set of songs where each one led into the next, thus creating a unified story. The lyrics weren't going to be nice and neat.

Gaye was known for singing about romance and love, not the realities of everyday life. After a listen through, Gordy had doubts about the album selling.

What is the risky album that Gaye was fighting his label for? It's none other than the game-changing and universally acclaimed *What's Going On*.

The album challenged and enlightened the listener, breaking the stereotypical mold of that time. It never would have happened without Gaye's deeply rooted belief in the album. This belief and persistence allowed future artists such as Stevie Wonder more creative freedom and independence on their albums.

This belief ultimately allowed him to push the boundaries again with the release of his album *Let's Get It On* (one of my favorite albums ever), which was a collection of strong and poetic erotic themes that weren't common in music at that time.

Ok, I bet you're wondering, "Is this a fitness book or a music history book"?

This example of a talented artist fighting for what he believed in is the perfect example of what's needed in your fitness journey. You must equip yourself with a bucketful of belief. You must be willing to go to battle every day for your goals and desires. Not only do you need to believe in what you're going after, but you need to believe you deserve whatever it is you desire.

Here's some quick food for thought: "If you don't deserve to build a body you can be proud of while living a fulfilling life, then who does?"

Knowing your mission (aka your "why") is crucial before starting your journey (strategy #1). There's a difference between being interested in a goal and being committed to it.

An interested person quits at the first sign of resistance (e.g., your record label trying to dissuade you or a stressful day at work leading you to settle for cookies). A committed person stands their ground and believes 100% in what they're fighting/going for (being persistent about an album until it finally happens or still going to the gym after that stressful day).

Meet the potential voice of impending doom

There's this nagging little voice inside our heads that tells us...

"You're not good enough." "You're going to fail (again)." "You can't do it."

"You need to stop before you feel any worse." "Fitness isn't for you."

"You're either born with the genes to be a fitness specimen or you'll just be an average Joe or Jane."

This (nagging) voice appears whenever you embark upon a new journey, whether it's losing weight, entering a relationship, starting a business, writing a book, recording an album, saving a city, or going after any other dream. The voice shows no mercy.

This (nagging) little voice's identity is self-doubt—the thing that kills our dreams. The thing that makes it (damn near) impossible to believe in ourselves. The thing that keeps us in bed paralyzed, and dreading facing the day. The thing that tells us we can't succeed with our fitness goals.

Self-doubt can, and will, destroy you if you let it. If anyone knows this...it's me.

Throughout most of my life, self-doubt has been my arch nemesis. Every corner I turn, it's waiting for me with open arms.

Lack of confidence with women. Fearful to write. Insecure about my body. Always needing to get leaner. Constantly searching for happiness (from all the wrong places). Seeking approval from others to determine my self-worth.

Sharing my words with the public—what would they think? On an off day, I'd think, "Oh, hell no" and I could lose my progress. With self-doubt controlling my life, it was impossible to live life as I desired.

What changed all of a sudden?

Belief. Simple. But powerful.

I started to believe. Even when things weren't 100% clear, I still believed. I persisted, even though on the inside, those steps were gut wrenching.

Seems simple, but changing your beliefs and initial thought patterns is a process that requires daily practice. That vision or dream you have about building the body you want and thriving at work will never be 100%

smooth sailing or filled with absolute certainty. Developing this mindset requires you to venture inside your internal world.

Reframe your mind

Our beliefs are everything. If you believe something to be true, you tend to search for things that support these truths and ignore everything else.

Your thoughts and pre-existing beliefs shape your feelings, which engineer your actions. Without awareness, your brain leaves you spinning your wheels. The way to defeat this is to reframe your approach and your initial thought processes.

Realize that self-doubt and fear never go away. How you handle them is what's important. This includes letting go of trying to be perfect (no such thing exists—this is procrastination in disguise and resistance at work).

Instead of telling yourself, "I'll never lose those fifteen pounds," realize those fifteen pounds won't disappear in one day. Focusing on losing fifteen pounds every day makes you anxious and disappointed because the goal hasn't come to fruition.

You'll never realize progress because you're fixated on the end goal instead of the process. Instead, make a personal pledge to commit to the process. Focus on the essential daily habits needed for that fifteen-pound loss to become a reality.

There is no time for waiting. The most important action for you to take is to start immediately and be intentional with your choices. Only give your energy to habits and actions that will provide value to your life and specific goals.

The first step in making a change is to believe you can have what you want.

Are you ready to take control?

If you're tired of feeling like a helpless victim at life, then stop—you're much stronger than you think.

If you're tired of telling yourself what you can't have, then stop—you can get whatever you go after (within reason and focus).

If you're tired of using lack of willpower and inspiration as an excuse for not going after what you want, then stop, make a plan, and take small steps each day to reach them.

If you're tired of telling yourself that weight loss isn't for you, then stop. It's not your genetics that's the problem—it's your lack of focus, lack of direction, and lack of positive habits.

Now...

It's time for you to believe in yourself. Show up even when you don't feel like it. Don't let fearful thoughts prevent you from taking action. You'll gain momentum and inspiration as you take action. Embrace any obstacles that head your way (there's opportunity within them). Your past setbacks aren't your present or your future.

You're in control. You have the ability to change anything you want. You have the power to create a better life for yourself. Your mind, career, body, and health are in your hands.

But everything starts with believing.

Robert Collier states that we can do "only what we think we can do. We can be only what we think we can be. We can have only what we think we can have. What we do, what we are, what we have, all depend upon what we think."

Change what you choose to believe in and change your expectations of yourself. Give yourself a new story arc.

Your mission, should you choose to accept:

Grab a sheet of paper or start a new document and type out some beliefs that are holding your fitness back. Once you have these beliefs written on paper, analyze each one and ask yourself, "Are these truly my beliefs, or have these beliefs been programmed into me by family, friends, peers, media, or any other external influence?"

You can't reprogram your mindset until you know exactly what you're thinking, why you're thinking it, and where this train of thought initiated from.

Strategy #3: Avoid the Tomorrow Concept & Start Now

"Until one is committed, there is hesitancy, the chance to draw back, always ineffectiveness. Concerning all acts of initiative (and creation), there is one elementary truth, the ignorance of which kills countless ideas and splendid plans: that the moment one definitely commits oneself, then Providence moves too.

All sorts of things occur to help one that would never otherwise have occurred. A whole stream of events issues from the decision, raising in one's favor all manner of unforeseen incidents and meetings and material assistance, which no man could have dreamed would have come his way. Whatever you can do, or dream you can do, begin it. Boldness has genius, power, and magic in it."

—W.H. Murray

"Once I have more time, I'll start working out; things are just too busy right now." "This is my last day of eating 'dirty foods'—it's all *'clean eating'* starting tomorrow."

"I'm going to hit the gym hard starting next week." "It's already Thursday, I'll start my diet fresh on Monday—you can't start a new diet in the middle of the week, right?"

"After this weekend, I'm going to be on my best behavior." "I have too many work projects this week to start eating healthier."

"My friends will give me crap if I order something healthier and don't indulge in drinking as we watch the game."

Blah, blah, blah...

The perfect time and place to begin is just a fantasy we concoct to delay taking action. Waiting for the perfect moment when all the stars align sounds like a damn good story in our heads.

Unfortunately, "Captain Reality" has different plans in store for us.

This isn't a Hollywood romantic comedy. Something will always be there to try to seduce you into waiting for another seemingly perfect moment.

If you wait until tomorrow, wait until next week, wait until work slows up, wait until you feel motivated, wait until the weather is favorable, wait until all your finances are in perfect order, wait until you received your promotion, wait until {any other excuse}—you'll still be waiting once whatever magical freeing moment you told yourself you'll finally be able to start arrives.

This moment is ultimately all there is. It's empowering to choose "now" to make a change. People who consistently wait until tomorrow and delay taking action just like the idea of making a commitment. It's nothing more than a Hallmark feel-good story for them.

At the end of the day, a desire to change is still only a desire until some kind of action takes place. Ripples won't be created in your life just because you want to change something. Ripples begin to manifest once you take action—any kind of action.

If you truly want something, and it's within your power to start, you'll begin as soon as possible, even if it isn't the right step or the prettiest step.

When you see that girl who takes your breath away, do you wait until tomorrow when you'll be wearing a newer shirt or next week when your work projects aren't stressful? Or do you simply say, "Hello" (not in a Lionel Richie tone, though I love that song)?

Odds are, if this girl is that mesmerizing, you'll say something—even if it's the nerdiest and cheesiest comment.

Fitness is no different. It's not important that you initially execute with precision and grace—it's important that you get off the sidelines and do something. Taking action is what delivers a world-class body. Taking action is how you can potentially land that dream date with the girl who astounded you.

As Gregg Krech in his wonderful must-read book *The Art of Taking Action* likes to remind us, "*Action isn't something that comes after figuring things out. Action is a way of figuring things out.*"

Your mission, should you choose to accept:

Start now on something. If you get confused or lost, it's not a big deal. Keep doing something and figure it out as you go along.

Strategy #4: Seek Antifragility in Fitness & Life

According to Naseem Taleb, author of *Antifragile: Things That Gain From Disorder,* there are three outcomes that can occur to an object if an earthquake occurs:

1. The object is hurt by the earthquake (fragile)

2. The object is unfazed by the event (robust)

3. The object gets better because of the event (antifragile)

How do earthquakes and these scenarios relate to fitness?

Simple.

Your ability to handle chaos and the random events of everyday life plays a pivotal role in how successful you will be with fitness.

A fragile person can't handle variation and needs to be handled with the utmost care. A fragile person falls off the fitness wagon if their normal workout time is interrupted, leading them to skip their training session. If they slip up on their diet early in the day, they'll most likely treat the day as if they're at the Golden Corral.

A robust person doesn't need to be treated with such delicacy. Variation to their day doesn't affect them. If things fall apart, they'll build themselves back up exactly how they were beforehand. What you see is what you get.

If randomness occurs throughout the day for the antifragile individual, they won't crack under pressure; they'll actually get stronger. Just as the mythical Hydra, as Taleb points out, becomes stronger: cut off one head and two heads will appear in its place. The human body is naturally antifragile—especially after you introduce strength training into the mix.

Think about it—you lift heavy objects (i.e., weights) and your joints, bones, and muscles rebuild themselves so they are stronger for the next time around, just in case you add extra heavy objects (i.e., more chaos into the situation).

Your body gets stronger by enduring uncomfortable and challenging situations. If you don't participate in any kind of strength training, your muscles, bones, and joints atrophy and become weaker because of the lack of chaos (i.e., weights/resistances) they are exposed to.

To engineer your desired body, you need exposure to randomness and the uncertainties of each day. Once you stop challenging yourself (your body in this case), your body starts to suffer as a result. Eliminating all discomforting situations from your life morphs you into a fragile individual.

Here are a couple of ways you can introduce antifragility into your fitness life.

1. Weekend events, birthday parties, happy hours with friends, date nights, or any special occasions

Solution: Have one free day per week where you allow yourself to indulge guilt-free. It's highly likely that at least once a week, you'll have some event, date, or social gathering where eating healthy is going to be difficult or not ideal. Rather than fight it and try to rely on willpower (an untrustworthy friend), embrace it and go with the flow. Indulge with zero guilts given.

This doesn't mean you have the green light to have a free-for-all on junk food—this is just allowing you some breathing room to enjoy your favorite foods while continuing in pursuit of your fitness goals.

Allowing this indulgence is beneficial psychologically and physiologically in the long run because no one wants to be the person who can't eat anything whenever they go out (that is no fun).

2. Strength training

Solution: Challenge yourself intensely with weights (with good form, so you stay safe) and use enough resistances with the weights (i.e., chaos) that it forces your body to rebuild stronger for the next time around.

By deadlifting, hip thrusting, and squatting challenging amounts, you're forcing your nervous system, joints, and muscles to adapt.

Don't do the same workout for months on end. Keep trying to improve in the gym. Track your workouts and improve on them. You could sprint a couple times a week and add a few more sprints or increase your distance (while staying safe) each week.

3. Everyday nutrition scenarios

Solution: If you rely on prepacked meals, cleanses, juicing, detoxes, Jenny Craig (is that still around?), Nutrisystem, microwave dinners (brave soul), or any other company food models, what happens if they disappear?

Most likely, this will cause a huge disturbance in your daily routine, thus crippling and hampering your fitness goals. All the above options are fragile solutions.

Here are a couple solutions to make your nutrition more antifragile:

- Learn how to cook (you control all the ingredients, ladies love it, you have options with foods, and you avoid relying on one company and/or person).
- Show no fear and try new foods (adding new items to your repertoire will train your taste buds to accept new flavors).
- Fast one day a week.
- Change up your meal frequency and daily caloric intake; eat more on workout days compared to non-lifting days.

The options are limitless. Just don't stay comfortable and cozy inside your warm and safe bubble called the comfort zone.

Your mission, should you choose to accept:

Pick one part of your fitness routine and throw some randomness into it, starting today.

Strategy #5: What *Lord of the Rings* Can Teach You About Embracing the Journey

When Frodo Baggins begins his journey, he doesn't consider himself heroic, nor would anyone with half a brain.

He isn't wise and powerful like the mighty Gandalf. He isn't a strong and mighty warrior like Aragorn. He isn't a superb archer like Legolas.

If you examine Frodo on the surface, he lacks every hero attribute.

Frodo is short, weak, indecisive, and immature, and he carelessly places himself in danger around every corner the group turns. The Frodo at the beginning of the journey couldn't carry out the mission at hand unless he evolved and morphed into something greater.

Only through the experiences of the journey did Frodo ultimately gain the courage and strength to destroy the ring and fulfill his mission. He's far from being the only one to undergo a transformation through a journey.

From Michael Jordan getting cut in high school basketball, Wilma Rudolph overcoming great odds to become a world-class sprinter, and Jackson Pollock continuing to paint despite the critics—one doesn't have to search far to notice that a person's journey often leads them to greatness.

What's the journey look like for you?

Any type of goal, mission, or event you're chasing after has its own specific journey encompassing a beginning, middle, and end.

The beginning (1% of the journey) – You have a desire to change. You feel some mystery force pulling you (wait a minute, am I talking about the force?). Perhaps this yearning to change involves losing fat, building muscle, or training for an event. Nevertheless, the journey starts by placing one foot on the ground and stepping forward (even if it's a baby step).

The middle (98% of the journey) – This is the meat and potatoes of the entire operation. This is where you acquire the necessary skills and knowledge to lose fat, build muscle, and learn how to keep it off for good (hence, shortcuts are a bad idea).

End (1%) – Frodo arrives at Mount Doom, destroys the ring, and then heads back home. The movie is over. We sat through three movies to watch him trek to the mountains and the ending is only 1% of the movie. (If you're into time, the ending lasted an estimated 15 minutes; please don't go back and try to prove me wrong.)

This isn't to downplay the ending because this is where you'll enjoy the fruits of your labor (e.g., losing those 15 pounds), but be aware that the ending is often not what you expect it to be.

Three beneficial things that happen as you go through the journey

Just as Frodo stumbled, cried, pouted on numerous occasions, and almost gave up, you'll at times question if fitness is for you and if you're strong enough to succeed.

You might pout or throw a three-minute pity party about why fitness isn't for you. No matter what you do, realize that going through the journey is pivotal, oftentimes ugly, and a necessity to becoming an improved version of yourself. As you go through your journey, these three attributes start to become a part of your identity.

1. You slowly start to morph and experience true change –We already know that the person you are at the beginning of the journey can't be the same person at the end of the journey if actual change is the goal.

At the beginning, change feels overwhelming and damn near impossible. However, through the journey, you'll learn that change is a gradual process that slowly happens—not something instantaneous. As you're losing weight, it'll often feel that nothing is happening, but over the course of weeks with consistent daily action, you're slowly creating a domino effect. This is where one event (i.e., a daily action toward your weight loss) will set off a succession of similar events, thus leading to large improvements over time.

2. You become wiser – You won't be Gandalf smart. But you'll become significantly wiser as you trek through your journey. While this specific journey is primarily focused on fitness, you'll quickly realize that the skills acquired through your fitness journey positively translate into other aspects of your life.

You'll learn to balance life and fitness, make better food choices, and have better relationships—all without losing your composure. Gaining experience and smarts brings about an inner confidence that you can achieve anything you set forth to do.

3. You'll learn that you're capable of 100x more than you thought was possible – If you would've told me in high school that I would be deadlifting 500lbs, benching over 300, and fluctuating between 190-200 pounds for the majority of the year, my afro-sporting, oversized-clothing-wearing, 160-pound baby-faced self would've fallen out of the chair laughing (and probably hurting myself in the process).

It's been over three years since I quit pursuing a medical education. If you would've told me that I would be sitting in cafes and parks writing and sharing articles on the Internet, I would have laughed at you while drinking a mojito (and pretending to be way cooler than I really am).

Even eight months ago, I wanted to write a book, but my fear was strong and my self-confidence was abysmal. I thought people who wrote books possessed something extra that I lacked. I thought they possessed special mutant abilities. I thought they were part of the X-Men, but I was wrong—they're just everyday people who show up each day and consistently do the necessary work for their goals.

At the beginning, Frodo never imagined performing these heroic feats. Along the journey, he discovered that inside of him lies someone with guts, heart, and determination. At the beginning, you might not be able to see clearly the body you want, how it will be done, or how you'll be able to manage all facets of what is going on in your life.

We've all experienced these same emotions, but starting the journey is about having the gusto to take action and believe in yourself.

Starting a fitness journey is difficult. Fitness is a skill, just as painting, writing, playing an instrument, and delivering a world-class speech are skills. It takes time to become skillful and things might get ugly, hazy, or scary along the way.

However, know that at the end of tunnel lies a person who will be

100x better at their craft and skill. The stories we play in our heads are mental barriers. We're our own worst enemies at times. We create invisible scripts stopping us in our tracks.

When you keep moving forward in your fitness journey, no matter the obstacles or how you feel, you develop character. These situations and moments are lessons. Just as Daniel from 'The Karate Kid' reflected and grew from those seemingly mundane and laborious chores into a worthy student of karate, reflect and grow from your situations and let those moments serve as your Mr. Miyagi ("wax on, wax off").

You're capable of so much more, but the potential only materializes if you get out of your head and embrace the journey to becoming a healthier version of yourself.

Your mission, should you choose to accept:

Identify what you're most worried about on your journey. Ask yourself if it's a valid worry, or if this is an invisible and ludicrous script created by the voices inside your head.

Strategy #6: How Newton's First Law of Motion Can Guide You to Success

"It does not matter how slowly you go, as long as you do not stop."

—Confucius

Back in the days of prepping for what I thought was going to be my career in medicine, I had to take a series of physics classes. In the physics world, momentum equals mass times velocity. The more mass and velocity an object has, the greater its momentum.

We go from being a body at rest to a body in motion.

Sir Isaac Newton's first law of motion states, "An object at rest stays at rest and an object in motion stays in motion with the same speed and in the same direction unless acted upon by some outside force."

Just like physics, our fitness goals have their very own momentum.

In physics, the larger the mass, the harder it is to get started. In fitness, the larger the mass (i.e., your initial step to getting started), the harder it is to begin your fitness habit.

Any time you set out for a goal and the first step requires too many steps for activation, initial momentum isn't generated. This subsequently leads many to quit due to little progress shown and confidence not developed.

I wanted to write a book, but the thought of writing so many words in a cohesive manner felt overwhelming at the beginning. When I started to learn how to salsa dance, I freaked out and ran to the bathroom for some deep breaths after watching the groups of men and women gracefully sliding across the dance floor. When I started strength training, I had visions of a lean and athletic 200 pounds, but 200 pounds was light years away from my initial weight of 165 pounds.

Whether it's writing a book, learning to salsa dance, or starting a fat loss goal, it's essential to get some small early wins. Initial small wins could be writing 250–500 words daily, learning the basic steps to salsa, or losing those initial three to five pounds.

These might seem trivial in the big picture of things, but the main objective is to get the ball rolling. That's all that matters. If the ball doesn't start rolling quickly enough for you to gain confidence and belief, you'll inevitably and logically quit.

Prevent this scenario from becoming a reality by making small daily commitments. As you continually go along, you'll start to gain more and more steam to further your progress. Confidence comes from doing, which is born through momentum.

To reiterate Mr. Newton's first law of motion, "The tendency of a body in motion is to keep moving; the tendency of a body at rest is to sit still." It's significantly easier to keep moving once you have some momentum than it is from a dead stop where momentum is nonexistent.

Some type of action needs execution each day to keep the momentum train rolling. It's easier to build a fitness habit with fifteen minutes of daily exercise than it is to sometimes exercise and sometimes become a couch potato.

Don't underestimate the power of one

One push-up, one squat, one email to someone who could hire you for your dream job, one email to a role model, one dance lesson, one phone call to that pretty lady, one healthy meal, one "no" when you normally would've said "yes," one paragraph toward that book, one brush stroke toward that painting—it all puts you one step closer to your ultimate goal.

It's easier to finish that book if you write words every day (even if some days it's significantly less than others). It's easier to learn that dance pattern when you practice every day for as little as fifteen minutes. It's easier to become more conscious of your food choices by focusing on one meal at a time.

Daily momentum buildups prevent you from falling into the inevitable sand traps that stick their rear ends out.

Confidence is given birth by momentum

What do a ladies' man, Batman, the Beatles, and Spider-Man have in common with individuals who have succeeded with fitness?

They all started their journey toward mastery by completing small daily activities.

A ladies' man initially might be scared to talk to women, but putting himself out there and saying hello to one girl a day helps him become more comfortable. Bruce Wayne becomes Batman, but he doesn't necessarily know if he's capable of becoming the legend we know him as until he places himself out there and nabs a couple of criminals.

The Beatles weren't a megahit initially; they created momentum and birthed confidence by playing in smaller shows and honing their skills.

Initially, Peter Parker wasn't the wisecracking superhero we know him as. He faced many moments of self-doubt and became the hero he is by taking daily actions and learning on the job, even though he wasn't necessarily ready for prime time.

Individuals in fitness became successful by taking it one workout at a time.

Look at your momentum as a snowball rolling down a hill. As the ball rolls along, it grows and picks up speed. Your fitness habit is the snowball. Start with one small commitment.

For example, eat one healthy meal per day and over time you'll start to notice that one healthy meal per day becomes two, then three, and so on.

Momentum manifests from doing—not obsessively planning or pretending to gain more information (procrastination in disguise). You'll never be 100% ready. The fear and uncertainty never vanish—you just learn to acknowledge the fear and the uncertainty and continue to move forward.

Little victories morph into large victories. Small accomplishments become large feats. One workout becomes a succession of workouts leading to a remarkable body.

Two simple steps for creating bulletproof momentum

1. Realize that momentum takes time to generate – You wouldn't expect to be able to run a marathon on day one. You wouldn't expect to become the next Hemingway and write a timeless classic on day one with no previous writing experience.

You wouldn't expect to paint the *Mona Lisa* on day one if you'd never painted before in your life. You wouldn't expect to become the next Arnold Schwarzenegger after one month of training.

Starting a fitness habit isn't any different. You shouldn't expect to jump into a rigorous program on the first day if the only exercise you previously did entailed going for "power walks." Stay realistic with your current conditioning levels. Assess where you stand and then base your fitness goals on that. If you're sedentary, pick a small achievable goal that is doable and gets the snowball rolling down the hill.

For those who are overly deconditioned, committing to daily walks is the perfect starting point. Challenge yourself, but don't overload your hard drive.

2. Carve out time every day (even if it's a few minutes) – Steven Pressfield has an excellent quote in which he states, "Our enemy is not lack of preparation; it's not the difficulty of the project or the state of the marketplace or the emptiness of our bank account.

The enemy is resistance. The enemy is our chattering brain, which, if we give it so much as a nanosecond, will start producing excuses, alibis, transparent self-justifications and a million reasons why he can't/shouldn't/ won't do what we know we need to do.

Start before you're ready."

It's easy to get lost in the busyness of our days and tell ourselves we'll start back tomorrow. It's easy to blame a creative project or work meeting for missing our gym session. But this is merely resistance at play.

Successful artists, musicians, writers, executives, and fitness enthusiasts show up every day. They don't wait for the muse or the magical beacon of inspiration to arrive. They create it themselves by doing something.

The secret for bulletproof momentum is frequency of the activity, not duration of the activity. Even if you can't make it to your regularly scheduled 45-minute strength-training session, that doesn't mean you should just sit in your office chair and mail it in for the day.

Squeeze in 15 to 20 minutes of activity by taking a walk or performing a basic bodyweight circuit.

As Pablo Picasso reminds us, "Inspiration exists, but it has to find you working." Go ahead and get that body in motion, no time for resting and "planning."

Your mission, should you choose to accept:

Take a baby step that feels effortless and almost too easy toward your specific fitness goal. What is your daily action that you'll take to continue your momentum?

Strategy #7: Don't Be Afraid of Failures, False Starts, & Setbacks

"You may encounter many defeats, but you must not be defeated. In fact, it may be necessary to encounter the defeats, so you can know who you are, what you can rise from, how you can still come out of it."

—Maya Angelou

There's this enchanting scene that exist in our minds. We fantasize about this idea. We tell our story to friends. We tell ourselves that once we get [insert your item], we'll be happy and all of our problems will vanish.

We work toward our goal. We place deadlines on when we should finish. We start to obsess over the goal and maybe let it consume us. We place all our faith on this moment and expectations that this will change everything.

Then, the day of reckoning arrives.

Our deadline passes and we didn't hit our expected goal. Whether due to work getting in the way, catching an illness, or some other related issue, our fitness goals weren't met. Now we're pouring ourselves a cup of self-defeat.

You expected this transformation to happen by a certain date, but it didn't happen. This must mean you're a failure. Maybe you've told yourself that it wasn't meant to be.

Why should you get back up? You've tried many times before with fitness. What's the point of trying again?

These are common questions and thought processes that many people (myself included, at one point) who struggle with fitness ask themselves.

Here's a (semi-fictitious) story

Raphael wants to get better with women and he starts to talk to women on a daily basis whenever he sees one that strikes his fancy.

He flirts with one girl at a coffee shop, one girl at the gym, and the other at the farmers market. The first two girls paid him no attention and rejected him. The third girl engaged him in conversation and eventually exchanged numbers with him. Due to him not getting down on himself after a couple nos, he now has a date this weekend.

In baseball terms, he's batting one for three, which is all-star level.

Cool story. But what's the point of hearing about Raphael's love life?

This is an example of persistence and reframing initial setbacks or moments of rejection into a positive. Raphael gathered information, implemented the useful feedback from the first two girls, and improved as he meet the third girl.

Your fitness exists under the same lens as Raphael's love life. One false start, two false starts, three false starts, or even ten false starts don't mean your fitness is forever cursed. This signals that you need to go back to the drawing board and figure out where you need improvement and where the trigger points of these false starts occur.

Whether it's losing weight, building muscle, earning a higher salary, becoming a skillful dancer, training for a marathon, building a business, fitting in your size-five jeans, or eating healthier, each of us have our own specific goals and challenges associated with them.

At one point or another, we've failed at one of our goals. Failing and hitting a couple speed bumps are a normal part of life. That's inevitable if you're trying to level up in this game we call life.

TV and marketing materials program us to think that overnight success stories are as frequent as a celebrity entering sex rehab (when did this become trendy?).

Unfortunately, this isn't real life (excluding the celebrity portion). These external outlets tell us what we want to hear instead of feeding us what we need to hear. If we allow external outlets to be the judge of our self-worth, then we're all going to feel like failures and less than human (due to the perfection spilled from these outlets).

Pay those stories no attention and operate under your own rules. There is no such thing as an overnight success story. All those characters in the overnight success stories and radical fitness transformations experienced many setbacks—there just wasn't a camera around to document these moments.

Think about it. What sells more? A feel-good story that you too can lose all your weight in 30 days without giving up your favorite foods or a realistic story about how losing weight will be filled with ups and downs and will potentially take months to achieve your goal?

Don't believe the hype. If it sounds too good to be true, it most likely is. Nothing valuable is obtainable through shortcuts.

Ok. Mini soapbox rant is over.

Setbacks and failures aren't permanent unless you allow them to be. Temporary setbacks and false starts toward your goals are necessary stepping-stones toward success. Failures are merely feedback that needs implementation as you continue along your journey. Setbacks are lessons, not dead ends.

Results might not have happened when you expected them to. You might've hit a couple of unexpected roadblocks along the way. Things may seem bleak for you.

That's life. Join the never-ending line of people who aren't in a perfectly controlled environment. One of the biggest lessons I've learned throughout these last few years is setbacks don't have to suck. Your setbacks don't determine your self-worth.

False starts and setbacks don't mean we need to:

- Live in shame

- Question ourselves

- Punish ourselves

- Feel hopeless

- Feel guilty

If your fat loss goal wasn't accomplished in eight weeks, like that magical $19.99 e-book promised you, it's not the end of the world.

If all your weight returns after that 30-day challenge, lesson learned. Don't chase Band-Aid solutions nor waterfalls (Idk, seemed appropriate).

If you're still not happy after completing that one-of-a-kind fourteen-day juice detox promising miracles, remember that magical elixirs can't replace hard work.

If your career isn't where you thought it would be now, there's plenty of story left in your book.

If you're not in the type of relationship you want, leave—there are plenty of fish in the ocean.

If you're still feeling lost and haven't found yourself, join the club.

It's ok. Take a breath (or two...or three).

Failures only manifest into your reality when you wave the white flag. Failures only become your identity when you stay down for the ten count after catching a right hook.

Your mission, should you choose to accept:

Put your detective hat on and investigate. Treat your setbacks as a mystery, a cold case, or pretend you're playing Clue.

Strategy #8: Willpower Isn't Your Friend

Have you ever stopped and thought about how many decisions you make on a daily basis?

If not, the answer is a metric ton (or close to 50,000). It's so many that, at times, you become drained just from having to make so many decisions. At times, thinking is exhausting.

We don't want to eat the cookies. We want to make healthier decisions. We want to go to sleep earlier. We want to start saying no to things that don't benefit our goals or add value to our lives.

Yet, we grab those cookies. Have that extra drink. Binge on that pint of ice cream. Miss our workouts. Stay up late at night watching Netflix and cruising Facebook (let's be honest, it's digital stalking for most of you).

What gives? Or, should I say, how does this happen?

Simple. There's this so-called friend of ours named willpower. Most people try to claim that through sheer willpower you can accomplish anything.

This is simply complete rubbish. Just as your car only has so much gas before running out and your light bulb only has so much energy before burning out, willpower, too, can run dry. Willpower is a finite resource that quickly burns out.

Our minds have this tendency to focus on the here and now and to hell with the future. It's about this moment and only this moment. When it comes to taking action, this could be helpful.

However, you see some cookies, you've been at work for eight hours, you're most likely tired and cranky—the cookies look really delicious now. You know you shouldn't have them, but now there are these voices sprouting up in your head telling you, "It's ok—it's only one." Then it becomes two, then five, but hey, you worked out three times this week.

This leads you down a slippery slope.

At 9 AM, you didn't want the cookies, but as you made more and more decisions throughout the day, you suffered from decision fatigue and had little energy left in the tank to say no again.

This is the same as having that friend you tell a secret to and they're not supposed to say anything, but eventually, after enough tugging from another friend, they spill all the information.

Willpower is the same. Once it's interrogated enough throughout the day (random daily life decisions), it caves in and betrays you.

What the heck is decision fatigue?

Decision fatigue refers to the fact that your decision-making ability will deteriorate over the course of the day. Just like your muscles fatigue during a workout, your decision muscles will fatigue as well after too much volume (i.e., daily minuscule decisions).

Every day, we make many decisions that require thought and in doing so, we steadily drain our willpower. A little decision here, a little one there, and you become less efficient at making the correct decisions on the big issues that matter most to your fitness.

You wake up and willpower is at 100%.

You have to think about what to wear (points deducted). You have to think about what you're going to eat (more energy being drained).

Now traffic is slammed, you're going to be late, you're already getting work emails, and the driver behind you is honking annoyingly—lots of energy depletion here. By the time you get to work, your stressful morning has your willpower already firing at half strength.

Now you have to think about what to eat at lunch, friends are texting you about their drama, coworkers are annoying—willpower is on life support now. You want something that is going to brighten up your day and add a little bit of pleasure (i.e., dopamine).

Cookies make their daily rounds at about 2:30 PM, and you can't say no this round because you just want to feel good and find something pleasurable (remember dopamine)—so you take the cookies.

You deserve it; your day has been stressful. Later on, you probably look back with regret and guilt for caving in. You may tell yourself, "I need to be stronger."

It's not your fault; you just didn't know any better. Willpower is conniving and sneakily charming.

But you can take measures to manage your willpower and cut its workload down by reducing your daily decisions.

Here are two easy areas to reduce the workload.

1. Make fewer decisions by cutting back on lesser ones such as:

- **Clothing choices** – Steve Jobs rocked black turtlenecks (I copied him, but wear black T-shirts instead). President Obama is either in a blue or gray suit. During the workweek, have your clothes ready the night before or on a simple rotation that requires little thought.

- When it comes to a night out on the town, then you can dress to impress.

2. Have a plan for exercising and eating

- **Know what exercises you're doing before you enter the gym** – Ideally, you should be on some type of training plan that helps you progressively overload throughout the weeks. This saves you time by keeping you from floating around and looking lost.

- **Know what you're going to eat** – Know your schedule for the next day and plan your eating times around your workload. Will you have to drink a shake or two due to extra meetings or longer work times? Will you have time to sit down and eat? If so, prepare a meal or two.

Make your day as automatic and simple as possible. Then you will have enough energy in the willpower reserve to make the right decisions on the most important things.

Your mission, should you choose to accept:

Pick one area of life where you could cut back on your minuscule decisions. Starting tomorrow, eliminate one minuscule step or task from your daily regimen. Preparation is your friend.

Strategy #9: Be Careful of Time Traveling

*"We all have our time machines, don't we. Those that take us back are memories...
And those that carry us forward, are dreams."*

—H.G. Wells

We all like to sit back with a tasty spirit, prop our feet up, and think about the good ole days or at least the days we thought were good.

Seldom do we live in the present moment. We're either wishing for different outcomes in the past, feeling regretful about the past, or holding onto some feelings from the past that we don't possess in the current moment.

When we're not revisiting our past, we're daydreaming our futures away and biting our nails about random events in the future that have yet to happen and most likely won't.

Time traveling is a dangerous game. While it provides helpful reminders of where we want to go and what we desire to accomplish, time traveling often creates unwarranted stories in our heads, which cripple us in the present moment.

We let past failures and preconceived notions stop us from taking action in the present. We daydream about a future where we have sculpted bodies along with the preconceived benefits that building the body of your desire includes.

The problem with both of these scenarios is that it takes you out of the present moment, which is the ultimate domino to constructing a future to your preference.

Unfortunately, Doc Brown and Marty McFly aren't coming to the rescue in their DeLorean to grant us the ability to travel in time.

Therefore, we have to do the next best thing, which is to let our past go and embrace the uncertainty of our future. If you struggled with fitness in the past, that's cemented and etched in stone. Obsessing over the past only brings about feelings of guilt, regret, and a bunch of "I should'ves." There is no time to play the "I should'ves" game. Just press play and focus on your "I musts."

The future is a crapshoot, full of uncertainty and guesses. Obsessing over the future brings about feelings of anxiousness and "I wishes." No time for wishes. Do or do not, but don't just sit there and hope and wish your heart away.

This leaves us with the present moment—the only moment that is moldable so you can wield it to your preference. Focusing on your present allows you to shape a future to your liking by taking the necessary action today to make that future a reality. Every single second, minute, hour, and day can and must be seized.

If you short-circuited in the past or quit your training program after a couple weeks, big deal.

Who cares? It's done and over with.

If you're sitting around in your chair daydreaming about your up-coming beach body that will make you irresistible to potential mates, but you haven't started consistently exercising or taking any initial steps for cleaning up your eating habits, call a time-out—you're getting way ahead of yourself.

Take it one day, one step, one workout, one meal, and one hour at a time and focus on ultimately winning the day in front of you. It's not sexy, but your rate of success is determined by your ability to execute on your mundane daily habits and behaviors.

Your mission, should you choose to accept:

Call a couple time-outs today. Set a reminder if that helps. Are you currently time traveling to the past or worrying and scripting some uncertain future event?

If so, give yourself a gentle reminder and bring yourself back to the present moment. What are some small but simple actions you can do today that can shape your future in a positive manner?

Strategy #10: Excuses Sound Best to Those Who Make Them

"To be successful in fitness, you need to have exceptional genetics." "You need to be in a perfectly conducive environment to achieve any type of fitness goals."

"Fat loss is only for the select few (i.e., everyone but me)."

"To be successful in the creative world, you have to be a natural at it and anything less is futile." "To be successful with women, you need to be rich and have an impressive portfolio."

"I'll never be a Hemingway." "A Picasso." A Van Gogh." "An O'Keefe." "A Michael Jackson." "A Prince." "A Bowie."

What's the point in even trying?

Surprisingly, many people sabotage all potential momentum with these fabricated stories before even stepping one foot onto the path toward achieving any type of goal.

This isn't fear so much as it's making excuses for not wanting to do the work.

We've all thought to ourselves...

"No, I can't do this, it's too hard." "I don't have enough experience; I need to read some more books before starting." "I don't have time at the moment to start, there's too much going on at work." "I'll look foolish doing this." "People might laugh at me for doing this." And the juggernaut, "I might fail."

When it comes to creating a fitness habit, procrastination and excuses come in different shapes, sizes, and news outlets.

These excuses are comfortable to roll around in. But buying fitness book number five isn't going to mean much if you haven't even taken action yet from the first four.

Watching another episode of a TV health program isn't going to make a difference if you haven't taken a single action from the previous episodes.

This is a common symptom of the information junkie—consume information 24/7, but never take action.

This person isn't learning. Deep down, this person is procrastinating and making himself feel better by telling himself he's researching a better plan, and then he'll start exercising. Most likely, this person's internal world is in chaos and he lacks confidence; therefore, he overcompensates in the external world with tasks to make himself feel like he has more control of the situation.

Ok, mini psychology lecture is over.

Excuses are a dime a dozen. Making excuses for why we aren't doing something sounds logical and acceptable in our heads (only because we're the ones blurting them out).

Excuses are seductive and sneaky. I'm sure there are people who've searched Google for a lifehack on solving the problem of making excuses. Unfortunately, just like most things in life, there aren't lifehacks to keep you from making excuses.

Not letting excuses rule your life comes down to acting with intent, displaying guts, and having the discipline to do the necessary work. Not letting excuses rule your life requires you to adopt a mindset of "doing what needs to be done" not "what you feel like doing."

Doing what you feel like doing is comfortable, cozy, and familiar—perfect ingredients for cooking up mediocrity and keeping the handlebar stuck in neutral while being eternally flustered and salty about pursuing difficult goals (especially fitness related ones).

Doing what you need to do births greatness and remarkability. You don't have to perform a big action; you just need a small action that slightly pushes you while making you slightly uncomfortable.

Excuses don't require a lifehack. Preventing excuses requires you be action oriented, regardless of feelings and circumstances. Simple as that. Unapologetically do it and own it.

If you want to train a certain way, do it unapologetically and wholeheartedly. If you want to eat a particular way or style, do it with zero regrets.

Just do it means you'll go for it and won't keep a spare in the reserves for just in case. Just do it means you won't let the "I's" of your ego stop you.

Once you have your vision, your why, and your direction, don't hesitate and let second thoughts hold you back.

Gregg Krech, author of *The Art of Taking Action: Lessons from Japanese Psychology* explains that there are three habits/excuses holding us back:

1. **Checking the list twice** – second-guessing ourselves

2. **Holding on** – hanging onto feelings about an interaction after it is completed (e.g., holding onto past fitness failures)

3. **Making a story in our heads** – taking someone else's word for something or reading into a situation and inventing a story about what those action/words/situations mean.

At the end of the day, to build the body you want and to thrive in life, work, and anything else, you have to take responsibility for your own actions. You are the captain of your own ship and can steer the vessel in any direction you deem worthy of exploration.

Your mission, should you choose to accept:

What's the biggest excuse you're holding onto at this present moment? What are you going to do about it? Write it down and refer to it when you're trying to slip back into your old excuses.

Better yet, after you write it down, hand it over to a friend or someone else who will keep you accountable.

Section III

Nutrition

You are what you eat. Garbage in, garbage out.

If you don't pay attention to what you're eating, then you're not going to have any results to show for your efforts. Oftentimes, you'll see people work their butts off in the gym day in and day out.

Months later, they look the same.

No matter what kind of training and however intense your workouts are, if you don't hone your nutritional craft and display some healthy behaviors and habits, you're not going to come close to building the body you want.

Just as you're a warrior in the gym slinging your weights around, make sure you're equally as intense when you're making decisions in the kitchen.

The next ten strategies are the core makeup to any successful nutritional program. We're going to uncover the true perfect diet. There won't be a nutritional lifehack plan revealed nor a strict, militant way of eating that labels fruit as evil or any other overzealous nutritional claim in the next ten strategies.

However, these ten strategies will give you the necessary tools to kickstart your nutritional habits. After reading over these strategies, it'll be up to you to test and assess which particular style works for you.

After all, each of us is a unique snowflake floating around in this universe. Enough blabbing. Let's dive into the basics of a successful nutrition plan for fitness.

Strategy #11: The True Identity of Food & Its Many Superpowers

"Let food be thy medicine and medicine be thy food"

—Hippocrates

We often think of food as this substance that makes our bodies lean, tight, and muscular. Food is often an afterthought, merely serving as a means to an end.

Eating is just something we do in order to survive and live as a species. Food, especially to hardcore fitness enthusiasts, is viewed as mere fuel. However, our bodies aren't a Ferrari or Lamborghini—food is so much more than this simplistic ideology.

Food provides energy to our bodies, but also includes micronutrients, water, zoochemicals, phytochemicals, and much more.

Without each of these components interacting with our bodies and providing for their functions, our bodies would suffer from an energy, performance, mood, and long-term optimal health standpoint. Food as just fuel is a simplistic nutritional tale that leaves out many essential details necessary to understanding the power of food.

Nutrition is more than just eating for aesthetics and becoming stronger in the gym. Nutrition affects every aspect of our lives for the better if we approach it with the right intention, approach, and attitude.

Food not only affects the outside of our bodies, it affects what goes on internally. While the outside gets all the acclaim and fame, the inside is what matters in the grand scheme of things. What goes on internally is ultimately what determines whether we'll thrive and prosper and live a quality life or become ridden with chronic disease and sickness.

Food is information and provides instructions for everything that goes on within our bodies. You are literally what you eat because that is the information you're feeding your body. Food is information to your genes, possessing the power to decide what genes turn off and on.

The way you look, feel, think, and age isn't predetermined but instead is dictated by what you choose to eat and drink on a daily basis. Food has the ability to help with...

- Decreasing stress
- Boosting your immune system
- Improving eyesight
- Lowering rates of depression
- Improving skin
- Regulating hormones
- Improving sleep
- Maintaining proper bone health
- Improving gut health
- Increasing concentration
- And many more gifts

Food is a drug that we don't need a prescription for. It is not something that needs to be consumed in secrecy. Food is the ultimate drug. It can act faster and influence our bodies better than any other drugs.

Food has the ability to bring friends, family, and strangers together in special ways. Food is immensely tasteful and pleasurable. It is not just something we transport around in a Tupperware container and mindlessly and begrudgingly consume. From the time it's a seed in the ground until the time it's fully sprouted and laid across our tables nourishing us and supporting our physique goals, food heals and connects people.

The first rule of nutrition is to appreciate food and see it as more than just a means to an end. See it as a gift. See it as something that heals you and your wounds. See it as a craft—a skill that someone put their time and energy into sharing and preparing for you.

Slow down while nourishing your body with nutrients. This not only provides a great moment to unwind, but to also express gratitude and take a break from the break-neck pace of everyday life. Take care of your body—you only get one of them. There are no do-overs or extra lives.

Your mission, should you choose to accept:

As you're eating today, slow down and take some time to show appreciation for the food you're consuming. A positive relationship with the food you consume lays a solid and sturdy nutritional foundation.

Strategy #12: Embrace Your Inner Dietary Scientist

While sitting in grade school, I daydreamed at times of putting the white coat on and becoming a scientist. From watching Bill Nye to conducting random chemistry experiments, I found science fascinating.

Most science experiments start in theory, and then you form a hypothesis to back up your rationale. Lastly, it's time to experiment. You have to test and test until you find the correct dosage for each variable in order to elicit the optimal result. Even the smallest of errors or mistakes in the dosage can throw off the entire experiment. While conducting the experiment, you're not 100% sure it's going to turn out as you expect.

Science is unpredictable and full of uncertainties. The only way to solve a problem or find a solution is to test and go back to the drawing board.

Countless dietary marketing machines preach that their dietary methods are superior, but our diets are nothing more than a chemistry experiment.

There are a plethora of diets and nutritional protocols in existence today, from Paleo to intermittent fasting to eating every two to three hours to "keeping the metabolism stoking." From warrior diets to Spartan diets to carb backloading to the Viking and Ninja diets (ok, I made those two up).

With so many diets breathing down our necks and spamming us at every corner, how are we supposed to know which diet is best?

What's the best diet for me? What's the diet that will get me lean and strong? Should I eat breakfast or skip? Will I lose muscle if I don't eat every two to three hours?

These are common questions when beginning a fitness journey toward specific physique goals.

Just like many things in life, nutrition isn't a black and white affair. The particular situation dictates the answer.

Ok, what is the perfect diet?

The perfect diet is the one that you'll stick to.

That's it? You've got to be kidding.

Sorry.

It's a giant letdown to those who wanted a magical one-size-fits-all answer that would sweep them away. Though there are many diets out there, nutrition is ultimately a choose-your-own-adventure (just like role-playing games). You possess 100% ownership over your diet.

There isn't a lifehack to your dieting. There isn't a magic wand that will erase your woes with one swift motion.

Just as a scientist puts his lab coat on and heads into the lab to mix and match chemicals until the perfect concoction formulates, you need to put your lab coat on to concoct your specific perfect diet.

The proven ingredients needed for a perfect diet (or as close to perfect as possible)

I said earlier that there isn't a perfect diet and that still holds true. There isn't a diet in existence that fits everyone's vibe and particular lifestyle.

There are particular ingredients that are essential to everyone's diet, but those ingredients come in different shapes, sizes, and amounts depending on the person. Your goal as a dietary scientist is to find a way of eating that supports your physique goals while seamlessly meshing with your individual lifestyle.

If you have to turn your life upside down in order for a diet to work, then you're on the wrong plan. The more your life is turned upside down because of fitness, the lower your percentages of succeeding due to the loss of your identity throughout the process.

Here are some questions to get you started toward concocting the perfect diet for you.

1. **What are my goals?** – Is it fat loss, performance, muscle gain, or general health? This is the easiest question to answer, but a necessary one so you know what you want to accomplish.

2. **How demanding is my job and what are some barriers it'll provide?** – A writer's daily regimen is different than a construction worker's. One has the ability to control their schedule and eat when they please, while the other is on their feet most of the day and meal frequency might be a little more difficult.

3. **Do I like multiple meals a day or just a few?** – Six perfectly portioned meals works just as well as three larger meals a day. I'm a little biased to eating fewer, more satiating meals due to my schedule and the pleasures of eating substantial meals. This is ultimately up to you to decide, but take into account whether you actually have the time to eat by the clock and whether that sounds pleasurable.

Your mission, should you choose to accept: it

Figure out your daily schedule and pick a particular way of eating for the week. Assess at the end of the week how it worked and then build from there.

Strategy #13: Don't put a Restraining Order on Your Macros

The blame game of always needing to find a scapegoat runs rampant in the fitness industry—particularly when the subject of nutrition arises.

Depending on which particular media outlets you follow, the unfortunate gurus you've been exposed to, and the dogma that's programmed into you, you most likely possess some slight biases and maybe even some fears toward particular groups of foods.

For the longest time, I was afraid of eating carbs and I religiously ate six to eight small, pre-portioned meals because I was afraid I wouldn't get results otherwise. I woke up in the middle of the night to down shakes at one point. However, at the end of the day, none of these actions was a necessity to obtain the body I desired.

Nutrition is a game that is user friendly and allows for customization to your liking (wait a minute; I just described the perfect video game).

In the 90s, we were living in the age of low fat, where fat was evil. Then we shifted toward embracing fat, pouring butter in everything (please stop with the butter in your coffee—there's nothing magical there) and blaming carbs for our obesity problems. Neither of those movements are the cause of our weight problems as a country.

One of our biggest weight problems comes down to an overall caloric game and, most important, a lack of the proper habits and behaviors. Struggles with weight are often due to a psychological issue that needs addressing. That won't be solved by another generic meal plan and being told to "eat this and eat that" or lame advice like "eat less and move more."

Each of your macros plays an essential role in developing a healthy, functioning physique. The best approach is to get each of these macronutrients in a proportional manner each day. Fitness isn't just about enhancing our outside appearance and ignoring our internal health.

You can look like a million bucks on the outside but look and feel like pennies on the inside.

A brief & not too sciencey introduction to your macros

Fats – Fats are damn tasty and can make any food delicious. However, some of the big and noteworthy attributes on the resume of fats is its role in regulating our hormones.

Fats provide insulation to keep our body temperature within normal range and cushioning to protect our organs. Fats are also essential for transporting fat-soluble vitamins such as vitamin A, D, E, & K throughout our bodies.

Carbs – Public enemy number one of the macronutrients. If you're like me, you've probably heard many times before that the reason why someone has a spare tire is because they're eating too many carbs.

May be true, but doubt it. That spare tire is there because they're eating too many calories in general and most likely not exercising. Carbs aren't part of the evil empire looking to destroy you. Carbs are delicious and essential to a properly functioning body and brain, and necessary if you want to have an excellent training session.

If carbs were evil and made people fat, then the Okinawans and the Kitavans would be some of the world's unhealthiest people due to the high percentage of their calories that come from carbs.

However, it's quite the opposite; those are some of the healthiest cultures in the world with the longest life spans to back it up.

Protein – Protein is a powerhouse that is oftentimes the favorite child of the three macronutrients. Besides being the basic building block of life, protein plays a vital role in providing healthy skin, hair, and nails, as well as in repairing our muscle tissues and cells.

Sometimes protein gets a bad reputation because of the excessive protein consumption of some bodybuilders and other competing athletes.

Everyday people aren't able to handle the copious amounts of protein that bodybuilders take in because we are not on vitamin S (steroids & other enhancers). People who aren't on vitamin S and are still ingesting copious amounts of protein are wasting money and most likely excreting the excess out.

Before you demonize a particular macronutrient or fall into a dietary cult where one macro becomes public enemy number one, remember that moderation is your friend and is usually the preferred path toward success. Extremes rarely win out or provide sustainable success. This journey is about the long haul, not just six weeks and then back to the status quo.

Your mission, should you choose to accept: it

Make it a goal to strike a balance with all three macros with your meals.

Strategy #14: Food Choices Come Before Anything Else

We might hop onto Google and look up the perfect diet, the optimal macronutrient ratio, various celebrity diets, supplements to melt our belly fat, and the optimal caloric formula for premium results.

However, before undergoing a nutritional exorcism, don't forget the basic ABCs of nutrition.

While it's important to know the basics of your macros and how to count calories, those sexy and exciting fitness metrics mean very little if you haven't addressed the most important issue of them all—your food choices.

At the end of the day, what you eat on a daily basis is the big determinant of whether you lose fat and build muscle.

Before ordering boxes of supplements, counting calories, figuring out your daily intake, or jumping aboard an online meal planning service, assess where you currently stand when it comes to your relationship with food. Specifically, take note and see what you eat on a daily basis.

If you're completely new to fitness, practice making better food decisions. Practice eating complete and balanced meals. Increase your daily veggie intake. Consistently eat your protein from quality sources.

Before counting calories or any other advanced nutritional tactic, know what each of your macros are and what kinds of foods belong in those groups.

Beginners and those who have inconsistent eating habits will do well to focus on making the correct food decisions first and foremost. As you're starting a fitness habit, it's essential you make your entry point as easy and seamless as possible. Knowledge of food is your greatest ally. Eventually you'll graduate up to counting macros and such, but even then, who wants to do that for the rest of their lives? That's why it's essential you home in on your basic fundamental levels of nutrition.

This allows you to eat intuitively and not freak out when you're at restaurants and hanging with friends and there isn't a macro chart for you to enter into MyFitnessPal.

Food choices before anything else. Get comfortable. When you take a music class, you don't immediately start flailing on the guitar. You learn to hold it properly, get used to its position, and learn where the cords are. Same with fitness and nutrition—get comfortable with your daily food choices and then gradually progress upwards.

Your mission, should you choose to accept: it

For the next couple of days, jot down everything you eat and analyze whether most of those choices are benefiting or slowing down your fitness goals. If it's the latter, focus on making good food choices before worrying about specific macro calculations.

Strategy #15: Everything Isn't Equal: A Tale of Why All Calories Aren't Created Equal

For fat loss to occur, we need to burn more calories than the body consumes. Before we go any further, let's define what a calorie is on its most basic level.

A calorie is simply a measure of energy.

Our bodies need energy to move, think, breathe, and to make sure our hearts continue to beat.

Unfortunately, in some circles, there's a simple belief about weight loss that states, "All calories are equal."

If only it could be that simple. Breaking the issue down to this simplistic model does a disservice to people trying to lose weight. This belief isn't taking into account the psychological, hormonal, and lifestyle influences and factors that play a role in obesity and ultimately our food behaviors.

Stating that all calories are equal is taking everything at face value and only looking at the numbers.

A 200-calorie container of cotton candy isn't the same as a 200-calorie protein bar. Different foods play different roles within our bodies and travel down different metabolic pathways based on their makeup (i.e., macros), which influences our fat loss and general health (most importantly).

I love candy and pastries, but a 2000-calorie diet consisting of Swedish Fish, root beer, "healthy" cereals, and cupcakes is going to be dramatically different than a 2000-calorie diet consisting of lean proteins, veggies, healthy fats, and sensible carbohydrate choices with the occasional pastry thrown in.

Focusing on just the numbers leaves out the effect foods have on our hormones and metabolism, as well as other internal health factors.

Let's think about our macronutrients, for example

Let's compare protein from a chicken breast to fructose, an energy source found in simple carbs such as candy and breakfast cereals (i.e., sugar).

Before going any further, I want to note that I'm not against sugar nor of the belief that sugar alone makes us fat, but I do realize that you can't exclusively eat pastries and expect to achieve optimal health.

Fructose enters the liver from the digestive tract, where it's then transformed into glucose and stored as glycogen. However, if the liver is full of glycogen, which is easily attainable, this excess turns into fat and ships out.

Consuming fructose in excess leads to insulin resistance and subsequently leads to fat gain over the long haul. Fructose doesn't register the same way as protein does with your body.

The body has to work harder to digest protein (think 30% more effort), and your body burns calories during this process. Calories from protein are also more satiating and don't lead to sugar spikes or hunger pangs the way eating the same number of calories from breakfast cereals would.

This simple example shows that a calorie isn't a calorie.

Different macronutrients affect your appetite in various ways. Fats are tastier and more filling as compared to simple carbs such as fruit. Think about calories from a chicken breast compared to calories from a chicken sandwich at your local fast-food joint. Foods loaded in trans fats can lead to inflammation, diabetes, cardiovascular problems, and cholesterol issues.

Just because you're trying to build the body you want doesn't mean you have to eliminate cake, cookies, and other favorites.

It does mean that you need to learn moderation and self-control.

Think of a ratio of 90/10.

Ninety percent of the time, you should choose foods that not only support your physique goals, but also positively support your general health and internal well-being.

Though we only see the outside appearance, what goes on inside is just as important. Keep the big picture in mind and eat for both optimal external and internal health. Providing your 90% is spot on, you can indulge for that 10% in whatever it is that you want.

Your mission, should you choose to accept: it

Evaluate your overall nutrition; are you eating at a 90/10 ratio? If not, think of one action you can take to start raising this percentage.

Strategy #16: Don't Go Chasing Sinkholes (Six of Them to be Exact)

From sinkholes that swallow cars, houses, and people sometimes (a cover-collapse sinkhole) to sinkholes that are shallow and span only a few feet across, often becoming a small pond (a cover-subsidence sinkhole), sinkholes affect our lives and environments in various ways, emotionally and physically.

Sinkholes and fitness are more similar than you think.

Just as sinkholes can become nagging thorns in our lives and provide obstacles of all shapes, your diet has the ability to engulf you into a black hole of frustration.

Macros are good, training is solid, but something is causing your momentum to come to a screeching halt.

We call these dietary sinkholes.

In an effort to save you from the devastating experience of falling into a sinkhole, here are six sinkholes to be aware of.

1. Having a hot & cold relationship with your diet

At the beginning of a relationship, you can't keep your hands off each other. Your love is on your mind 24/7. You hear a song on Spotify or see a particular flower, and you think of them. Your friend unknowingly mentions a word that reminds you of her, and you randomly start daydreaming of their appearance. The love is at an all-time high.

Next week, this person is annoying. You don't want to touch them, you're bickering over minute tasks, and you're complaining about their laziness with friends over a glass of wine. Being stranded in Siberia sounds infinitely better than being in the same room with them.

Sound familiar?

One minute you're counting macros to a tee, working out as if you're a Spartan warrior, sleeping like a good boy, and staying away from the booze and office cookies.

The next minute, you're taking the day off with your diet (after all, a couple days of relaxed eating won't hurt). You take rest days at the gym for "recovery purposes and to avoid overtraining." You plan to catch up on sleep over the weekend. You tell yourself a couple drinks won't hurt and that it's rude to say no to office cookies (plus you deserve to eat the cookies).

Just as hot and cold relationships never develop into anything of worth, following your diet in spurts isn't going to lead you to your desired results.

Your diet isn't a one-night stand. Your diet isn't a 3 AM last call option at the bar where anything will suffice. Your diet isn't a mistress. Your diet needs to be treated like royalty. Your diet is the love of your life. Nurture it. Work on it and keep it fresh or you'll be headed for a nasty split and that never ends well.

Most people see their diets as something with a start date and a specific end date. We as a society have a tendency to want things immediately and with as little effort and struggle as possible.

We'll cut carbs for six weeks to lose inches as fast as possible. We'll opt for a 30-day shred plan if it promises us all our fitness woes will be solved. Those methods yield few long-term benefits in terms of learning proper healthy habits.

Instead of approaching your health cyclically, find an approach that works year round. View your dieting as a lifestyle change, not just a brief period of changes.

2. Letting healthy buzzwords seduce you

I've been seduced more times than I care to admit. I'm a sucker for a good story, pretty face, nice collection of words, pretty combination of colors on the wall, or basically just anything that mentally stimulates me (I believe this is called being a sapiosexual).

This sounds familiar as well.

Fat-free. Sugar-free. Organic. Free range. Natural. Reduced sodium. Extra antioxidants. Feel free to add the other hundreds of buzzwords that go along here.

Buzzwords are trendy. Buzzwords are sexy. Your coworkers rave about these buzzwords as they attempt their latest health binge. Being seduced by trendy buzzwords is the same as chasing the magic pill that eradicates all our worries, fears, and problems and leads us to a utopia.

The best way to prevent unnecessary seduction in any situation in life is to be aware. Know what's going on. Seduction needs to reside behind closed doors and stay between the sheets, not show up while you're shopping down aisle five.

No matter if it's sugar-free, fat-free, or any other free—they still have calories in them.

Fruit is still fruit. Sauces are still sauces. Dressings are still dressings. Organic Oreos are still cookies. Baked Ruffles are still chips that are processed. Organic fried chicken is still chicken that's fried. Cereal is still cereal. Calories are still calories, no matter what the label states. Just because something is labeled organic or natural doesn't mean it's healthy. Your metabolism and hormones don't know the difference between organic and non-organic high-fructose corn syrup.

Just because the foods have trendy healthy buzzwords included doesn't grant you license to eat everything.

3. Dietary silent assassins

An assassin is noted for being stealthy, precise, and efficient.

While in the dietary world, you don't have to worry about a ninja slashing you physically, you do have to worry about a dietary ninja discreetly slashing your progress. Without awareness of this ninja, your fitness progress will never get on the right track.

What is a dietary assassin?

It is any type of food that seems unassuming to the average eye but is loaded with calories.

From calorie-loaded condiments to salad dressings, food additives, creams, and other decadent dressings for our coffee, these secret calorie bombs bring your progress to a halt if you're unknowingly using them throughout the day.

While creams, dressings, and other items aren't evil and don't deserve to be blacklisted, they still count toward your daily intake. The creams and syrups you liberally pour into your coffee still count as calories.

A little bit of cream won't cause a dent in your progress. But if you need sugars, creams, syrups, and various other items in your drink, let's be honest—you aren't a true coffee drinker and need to find a new caffeine source. What you're drinking sounds more like a caffeinated milkshake than a coffee.

Oftentimes, salads at restaurants have upwards of 800 calories, which is huge for a salad. Your caloric intake for salads shouldn't mirror your main dish. Sometimes the little things are stopping the engine from running on all cylinders. Be aware of the small calorie assassins going into your foods.

4. Not eating enough

"If I eat less food, then I'll lose weight more quickly." "I'm skipping dinner and not eating much fat with my food." "I'm skipping carbs." "Maybe, I'll just eat once a day."

Unfortunately, none of these scenarios leads to quicker fat loss. In actuality, these scenarios most often prevent you from building the body you want due to various physiological and hormonal factors.

Your body eventually catches on and starts to conserve energy. This leads to a slew of negative metabolic changes within the body. A couple of metabolic changes within the body that will occur are...

Thyroid production slows – Our thyroid hormones (mainly T3 & T4) are responsible for the metabolism of protein, fats, and carbs among a slew of other tasks. Thyroid output slows down if the body isn't getting enough energy. This preventative step is taken in order to maintain an energy balance, allowing you to function properly.

Muscle mass decreases – Maintaining muscle requires calories (as they say, "These muscle aren't going to feed themselves").

Your body, one way or another, will find a way to supply itself with the necessary components for energy. Our bodies crave fat and need fat for survival (especially our organs), so when worst comes to worst and our bodies aren't getting enough nutrients for energy, muscle is forcibly nominated as the first tribune for sacrificial purposes (i.e., muscles wasting).

Leptin levels decrease – Leptin plays a leading role as your satiety hormone. This hormone is produced in our fat cells and is designed to inform our brain that we have enough fat and we don't need to eat at this time. However, leptin's main job is regulating our energy balance—the amount of calories we expend and eat.

Leptin is an air traffic signaler relaying directions to your brain. High leptin levels relay to us that it's okay to stop eating. Levels on the low end ignite us to eat more since energy is needed.

In an overly calorie-restricted environment, leptin levels plummet while hunger levels increase and metabolism slows, thus causing you to burn fewer calories.

Testosterone levels slide down the drain – Testosterone is crucial to a properly functioning body for both men and women. This hormone is far from just being important to the bros. Extreme calorie restriction lowers your testosterone levels, decreases sex drive (not cool), and makes building muscle next to impossible.

Energy levels drop– From lack of motivation to a foggy brain to a sluggish body, a lack of calories will have your body whispering to take it easy and slow down. Good luck producing great workouts and thriving at work when you feel like the walking dead.

When you're trying to lose fat, eat as much as you can while steadily making progress. Only lower your calories once progress has stagnated.

5. Turning the weekends into an extravaganza

Monday through Friday, you're the perfect fitness soldier, but then the weekend comes and all hell breaks loose. From social gatherings to random temptations, the weekends are dangerous to those who aren't mindful of their actions.

Saturdays and Sundays are the same as the weekdays, besides maybe sleeping in later.

While it's okay to indulge with zero guilts given a couple times each week, it's not okay to relax every weekend and eat whatever you want and start back fresh on Monday. This approach is a great way to stall your progress. Don't place such tight restraints on your diet that when you indulge, it turns into an all-you-can-eat food festival.

6. Letting your diet stealthily become the ruler of your life

Are you declining invitations and hangouts with friends more frequently due to worrying about your diet? Are you thinking about food 24/7? Are you asking about macros while downing sushi or some massaman curry?

If every decision you think about comes along with "how will this affect my diet" or "does this fit in my macros," then you need to reel the situation back to a more reasonable and logical position.

A six-pack isn't worth trading in the life you once knew.

Your mission, should you choose to accept: it

Are you guilty of falling into one of the sinkholes? If so, take this week to escape your sinkhole and turn it into a strength. Remember, don't go chasing sinkholes (wait a minute, I thought it was waterfalls).

Strategy #17: Lose the Guilt (It's Not Worth It)

At times, the notion of healthy eating can start to consume us, especially those new to fitness. Food guilt possesses the power to psychologically paralyze us and, in extreme cases, lead to eating disorders and body image issues. Food guilt becomes a huge inconvenience in our lives and starts to affect our relationships, quality of life, and how we choose to operate on a daily basis.

The notion of "eating clean" can become a borderline obsessive issue.

Let's take a trip back into time and visit young Julian.

For the first few years of my fitness journey, I was a slave to hardcore fitness concepts and deeply entrenched in a narrow mindset about fitness.

From hardcore sessions in the gym to being a total fitness snob toward those who didn't agree with my principles of what training and nutrition should look like, I was a pawn to fitness. I tooted my own horn and worshipped obnoxious clichés and bro-science philosophies like, "Eat clean, train dirty," "Eat within 30 minutes of a workout," "Eat six meals a day to stoke the metabolism," and "Eat every two to three hours or risk losing your gains."

I even woke up in the middle of the night to take a casein shake in fear of going catabolic (i.e., losing muscle).

My intense desire for perfection controlled my emotions, behaviors, and thoughts. From eating disgusting and smelly tuna packets in between classes to walking around with measured portions of almonds and rice, I left nothing to chance.

This obsessiveness was in the best interest of my fitness, or so I initially thought. After all, I was seeing results, even if I was an emotional and lonely train wreck. If the pros and the hardcore elite in the fitness magazines carried around plastic food containers and coolers, then dammit, I'm joining team Tupperware as well.

Social life? Who cares. I'll party and date when I'm leaner. Plus, the ladies will flock to me once my biceps are bigger (this turned out to be a lie). Cheat days? Is this a troll or joke? No way, I'm not ruining my six-pack for one day of pleasure.

Committing a single mistake equated to me failing the day. I eventually let food guilt turn me into a recluse. I couldn't ruin my diet if I avoided social situations and stayed close to my fridge. It took a lot of time and effort to remove the stains that "clean eating" stamped onto my life.

In an effort to prevent you from following this path and letting "clean eating" seep it's discreetly poisonous fangs into your life, I've laid out four strategies to avoid letting food remorse dictate your life. After all, you're in control, not your diet. Mistakes and indulgences happen; we're human, not robotic.

1. Acknowledge, accept, and move on from your brief dieting mishaps

There's a reason that acknowledgment and acceptance are the first few steps toward any program, whether it's a broken heart, loss of a loved one, or recovering from an addiction. Acknowledging and accepting humbles and exposes us to our imperfections as humans.

And that's okay and 100% needed.

Mishaps often occur due to people following restrictive diets with no flexibility installed within the plan. Our diets are not a blood pressure machine at the local drugstore that needs to squeeze the life out of us in order to gather results.

Maybe you've been in my situation where you go out with friends and have one too many drinks or dip your hands in the chips and salsa a couple times too many.

The next day, you're feeling bloated. You feel all your efforts have unraveled because you had fun at the expense of keeping it clean with your macros.

It's going to be okay. Life happens. After all, what's the point of leveling up your fitness if you have to stay in dietary confinement to net results?

That's not cool.

Realize that one random night is minuscule in the grand scheme of things. Achieving progress with your fitness is about approaching it with the big picture in mind, not operating from a moment-to-moment standpoint.

2. Realize that perfectionism is only in fairy tales

I love fantasies. I especially love romantic comedies. So much so that it oftentimes leaves me with unrealistic dating expectations (thanks a lot Billy Crystal, Meg Ryan, Tom Hanks, and many others).

Often times, we have this pristine perfect little person floating in our heads that does 'x & x thing' flawlessly. Captain Reality arrives with a vengeance and shows us that this person in our heads has no chance of manifesting. The only time perfectionism happens is when the person never takes action. All the action takes place inside their heads; therefore, it stands no chance of ever being ruined.

Nobody is perfect. I'm certainly not perfect. Those fitness professionals, models, your CrossFit buddy who never stops talking about his WOD (workout of the day), and those everyday-selfie-taking Instagram models—they all make mistakes and occasionally fall off the fitness wagon.

Many successful people in fitness have experienced a plethora of false starts with revving their fitness engines up. If they tell you anything differently, they're lying. Perfection is about as likely as domesticating a unicorn.

Be kind to yourself. Forgive yourself. If you can show forgiveness to others and tell them it's going to be okay, why not give the same treatment to the one who matters the most—yourself.

3. Do or do not. There is no try with indulgence

If you're going to "cheat" on your diet, just do it and move on instead of letting it preoccupy your entire day. Your brain only has so much daily bandwidth. Use it wisely.

Cheating is 100% of the time associated with negativity, whether it's cheating on your partner, on exams, or in sport. Cheating is something forbidden, something that shouldn't be taking place, something that needs to be taken care of in secrecy—no one is supposed to know. Cheating is oftentimes used to make ourselves or someone else feel bad about something.

Saying that we are "cheating" on our diets means that we aren't allowed to do this or we shouldn't do this. Cheating brings shame, guilt, and stress as a tag-team partner.

Healthy eating doesn't need either of those characteristics. Healthy eating is eating in a way that satisfies your palate, supports your fitness goals, and helps you build the body you want while you enjoy the awesomeness of life. Healthy eating is about finding happiness and balance in the way you approach nutrition from a physique and pleasure standpoint.

Instead of cheating—indulge. Indulge with pride, enjoyment, and mindfulness rather than cheating in secrecy with guilt, shame, and stress.

Your mission, should you choose to accept: it

Are you currently guilting yourself about an issue? If so, let it go (brush it off your shoulders). Challenge yourself to indulge without shame and remove the concept of cheating from your vocabulary and life.

Strategy #18: Don't let Your Emotions Control Your Eating Habits

Our emotions either catapult us to greatness or drag us down into frustration and hopelessness.

When it comes to nutrition, this is true to the thousandth degree. From the stress of work, the pressure we feel from our friends and peers, or just plain boredom—there are plenty of reasons to fall off our diets.

Often, this takes the form of mindless eating, which occurs when we're eating without thinking about what we're doing. We're letting our external environments and our preconceived notions about what we're supposed to do control our eating habits. These notions and external stimuli don't have the slightest interest in our fitness goals.

One of the biggest elephants in the room is stress eating.

Do you constantly graze on whatever you see at the office (especially after seeing the morning reports)? Do you find yourself binging on chocolate after checking up on your latest freelance projects, emails, and designs? Do you find yourself snacking after family and friends stress you out with their problems?

Stress is an emotional vortex that sucks you into another dimension and leaves you in disarray.

Unfortunately, your problems with stress can't be covered up with money or resolved by the latest self-help books. And they won't be resolved by becoming more militant and restrictive with your diet.

The only cure for stress eating lies within. The cure comes down to honing your daily habits and behaviors. It requires that you become aware and practice slowing down (something that is difficult at times to do in America). To help you get on top of your emotions, here are a couple strategies to enlist.

1. Sleep – You'll soon discover that many issues in health and fitness revolve around getting quality sleep. Sleep is one of the cornerstones of fitness and without it, you've handicapped yourself before entering the ring.

Not focusing on your sleep is the same as entering a ring with Muhammad Ali and trying to fight with one hand—you have no chance of success. Sleep influences your daily food behaviors and decisions. Less sleep and that dollar pizza looks awfully enticing compared to a chicken breast.

Not paying attention to sleep raises your cortisol levels, thus decreasing the rate of your fat loss. Not giving sleep the respect it deserves helps you add extra layers of armor to your body (and we're not talking about clothes here).

2. Find pleasure in anything else besides food – Food is awesome, I get it, but not everything in life needs to be celebrated over food.

Promotion at work, you aced an exam, you got a girlfriend finally, or you just feel sad—so let's just eat something. You're bored, it's Saturday night, and your friends are lame and don't want to be social, so you do the next logical option—Netflix and chocolate cupcake ice cream.

Each of these food justifications programs your brain to associate food (often sweets, fattening foods, and copious amounts of booze) with pleasure and other addictive emotions. Boredom and loneliness work the same way, as we eat to pass the time or keep ourselves busy. Instead of eating just because, use these moments to gain some new skills, get lost in a book, catch up with a friend over a walk, or go on a date to the local museum.

3. Slow down – When's the last time you sat down and just focused on eating and appreciating the meal at hand?

Go ahead...I'll wait.

Odds are it took you a long time to remember. We live in the age of distractions and busyness. Put the brakes on; your food isn't running off the plate.

4. Discover your trigger points – Thich Nhat Hanh wonderfully states, "*Sometimes we eat, but we aren't thinking of our food. We're thinking of the past or the future or mulling over some worry or anxiety again and again. Don't chew your worries, your fear, or your anger. If you chew your planning and your anxiety, it's difficult to feel grateful for each piece of food. Just chew your food.*"

Let go of thinking about work and personal stress, and just take in the moment of enjoying the food. We all have different stories, scenarios, and environments that elicit the worst in us. It's imperative we discover what those are so we become aware when danger strikes.

Look at this skill as developing your Spidey sense for upcoming temptations. Is yours family, friends, significant others, work emails, work projects, the uncertain future you might have about your startup, or the thought of running out of material as an artist?

Whatever it is, the only way to defeat these triggers is to identify them so you're prepared. This helps you locate the source of your stress. Build this awareness by noticing your moods and thoughts as you give in to tempting foods and drinks.

At work, we're eating on the run, in the car, or while sitting in meetings. At home, we're watching TV, playing video games, stalking someone on Facebook, or daydreaming away on Instagram. It's never just about the food.

At restaurants, we're often distracted by our smartphones instead of being focused on our company. Our minds are racing a million miles per hour and food is an afterthought. It's just another task in the day instead of a highlight.

Contrary to what your work or the media tells you, multitasking doesn't make you more productive. It actually makes you less productive, unless you're in the 2% of the population that succeeds at multitasking according to researchers. But let's not lie: you're not in that group and neither am I.

Focus on one thing at a time. When it's time to eat, focus on the food. Sit down if you can and appreciate and savor the flavor of delicious foods. If you can't sit down, at least give yourself a minute or two to appreciate the food you have.

Your mission, should you choose to accept: it

Take notice of why you're eating. Are you hungry or just need something to do? Ask yourself this question each time you eat over the next few days.

Strategy #19: It's Not Always about the Best Actresses & Actors

In the fitness world, people are always (annoyingly) debating about the optimal protein ratios, which carbohydrates will make us sexy, the exact angle for maximum chest recruitment, who has a better lat spread, why fats are supreme, the optimal macronutrient balance – but, we often forget the little guys.

While the big three hog the spotlight, it's our micronutrients that are often the deciding factor in whether we will display a healthy body that isn't just an aesthetic marvel but that functions optimally as well.

After all, longevity and quality of life are vastly more important than displaying "hot abs" but feeling like three-week – old dog poop. What's the point of having a body that looks like a Ferrari when it performs like a 93 Chevy Malibu? Looks can only take you so far.

Just as supporting actors are important to movies, micronutrients are vital if you want a healthy, sexy, and high-performing body. Would *The Dark Knight* be as memorable without Heath Ledger as the Joker? Of course not. The same is true for the "supporting" nutrients.

It's important to keep up with our big three macros (main actors), but remember that your micronutrients (supporting cast) are ultimately what is going to deliver an Academy-Award worthy film (your physique) instead of one that earns a Razzie award (a body that doesn't perform or function adequately).

Let's take a brief, but broad tour of our micronutrients so you can ensure yourself of earning an Oscar instead of a Razzie.

What are micronutrients?

You can view micronutrients as the silent machinery that propels your engine to function properly on all cylinders. Micronutrients play a vital role in a healthy functioning metabolism, the prevention and treatment of various diseases and health conditions, and the optimization of our health so we can perform at a peak state—mentally, emotionally, and physically.

Micronutrients are broken down into two types: vitamins and minerals.

A brief (and broad) primer on vitamins

Vitamins are broken down into water-soluble and fat-soluble vitamins. The big difference between these is that water-soluble vitamins are easily lost through bodily fluids; thus they need daily replenishment. Fat-soluble vitamins need dietary fats to help with the absorption process and aren't as easily wasted as the water-soluble vitamins.

A quick blurb on water-soluble vitamins

Not to get too scientific, but many of the water-soluble vitamins are involved with various chemical reactions within the body, as are other micronutrients. These water-soluble vitamins play a role in the metabolism of carbohydrates, proteins, and fat; assist in DNA synthesis; and acts as an antioxidant, to name a few of the responsibilities.

Your water-soluble vitamins include your eight B vitamins (B1, B2, B3, B5, B6, B12, Biotin, Folate [folic acid]) and vitamin C. Of those, vitamins B6, B12, and C are probably the most known and popular ones.

Vitamin B6 (pyridoxine, pyridoxal, & pyridoxamine) – Helps with protein and carbohydrate metabolism as well as assisting in blood cell synthesis. An easy way to get B6 is consumption of beef, poultry, and chickpeas.

Vitamin B12 (Cobalamin) – Helps in the metabolism of folate along with protecting our myelin sheaths (a coating that surrounds and protects our nerve fibers). This is the vitamin that vegans have difficulty ingesting naturally, since B12 isn't found in foods of vegetable origin. B12 is found in fish, poultry, dairy, and beef.

Vitamin C –An antioxidant that boosts our immune system, among a slew of other responsibilities. Look to your fruits and veggies, including potatoes, as great sources for vitamin C.

A quick blurb on fat-soluble vitamins

Vitamin A – Helps with our vision, immune system functioning, bone health, and our reproductive system processing. A couple sources include sweet potatoes, dark leafy greens, liver, fish, and carrots.

Vitamin D – One of its biggest roles is supporting proper bone health. The best way to obtain vitamin D is sunlight. But those of us who live in cloudy environments or refuse to step outside during scorching southern summer months (this is me) can look to fatty fish sources, nuts, egg yolks, and beef liver to name a few.

Vitamin E – An antioxidant that protects your body from substances called free radicals. These free radicals pose harm to your cells, organs, and tissues (this plays a huge role with our aging process). Look to seeds, greens, and nuts as quality sources of this vitamin.

Vitamin K – Plays a starring role in bone formation along with blood clotting. Vitamin K is found in leafy greens, spinach, and broccoli, to name a few sources.

A brief (and broad) primer on minerals

Just like vitamins, minerals are divided into two groups: macro (major) minerals and micro (trace) minerals.

A quick blurb on macro (major) minerals

Macro minerals are needed in larger quantities than the micro minerals. The more common macro minerals are:

Calcium – Pivotal role in muscle contractions and nerve transmission, and a huge component of our bones and teeth. While dairy is the most popular source of calcium, kale, turnip greens, seafood, and bok choy contain decent amounts as well.

Magnesium – Helps with muscle contraction and relaxation, and blood clotting, and assists our enzymes in over 300 chemical reactions that I will mercifully not recite. Look to leafy greens, potatoes, nuts, and seeds as your sources for magnesium.

Phosphorus – This mineral helps the body make ATP (this is what gives your body its energy) along with playing the role of a sidekick when assisting calcium to form our bones and teeth. This mineral is easy to find and deficiencies are rare; this food is found in meats, eggs, and nuts.

Sodium – One of the most vital minerals due to its association with regulating blood pressure. This mineral helps provide a balance of fluids within our bodies and is also important when it comes to muscle contractions (and therefore our performance in the gym) and transmission of our nerve signals. Sodium is in practically every type of food and is found in large quantities in processed foods.

Potassium – This is ying to sodium's yang. A diet rich in potassium helps offset the overconsumption of sodium found in many of our daily diets. Obtaining this mineral is relatively easy. Look to sources such as fruits, vegetables, sweet potatoes, and leafy greens.

A quick blurb on micro (trace) minerals

While the list below isn't comprehensive, it's a highlight of the more common and important trace minerals.

Iron – This is a complicated mineral that would take a long time to fully discuss. For simplicity's sake, let's just name a couple of the important functions for this mineral: essential for the production of red blood cells, carries oxygen throughout the body and thus helps our muscles store and use this oxygen, supports the immune system, and is involved with the development of the brain and nervous system.

The best sources of iron that are easy to digest are eggs, liver, lean red meats, salmon, oysters, and chicken. Other notable sources are kale, broccoli, spinach, and almonds.

Chromium – Mainly known for enhancing the effects of insulin. Excellent sources of this mineral are dark chocolate and nuts.

Iodine – This mineral is essential to maintaining a properly functioning thyroid. (I also like the way the word sounds.)

Why is a functioning thyroid important?

Your thyroid is the major player when it comes to regulating your metabolism and body temperature. If your thyroid isn't functioning optimally, that sluggish metabolism leads to a host of issues, with slow fat loss being one of them. Since the introduction of iodized salt, deficiencies haven't been as prevalent in the western world as they once were (just don't go overboard).

Good iodine sources are fish, potatoes, and iodized salt (of course).

Zinc – This might be my favorite micronutrient. Zinc plays a role in providing us optimal performance in the gym, improves energy levels and sleep quality, supports the male and female reproductive systems, and supports our immune system.

The highest sources of zinc are oysters, beef, and cashews.

A closing ceremony to wrap this lecture up

While the information may have seemed tedious or overwhelming, don't let either feeling deter you. You don't need to become obsessed with eating a food specifically for each and every mineral and vitamin on a daily basis.

- What this means however, is that eating an intelligent diet with each macro represented in an adequate manner along with a vast array of veggies is important for optimal health. After all, food isn't just fuel for our workouts; it's also a powerful form of medicine with each micronutrient serving an important role in achieving optimal health.

- While most foods are dominant in a particular nutrient or two, they most often include other nutrients as well in an adequate amount that will cover your daily requirements.

Your mission, should you choose to accept: it

Build your palate up by trying new foods weekly. Pick one or two new vegetables or fruits to try as an attempt to cover your daily micronutrient ratios.

Strategy #20: Supplements Can't Cover a Flesh Wound

Take this supplement and gain 15 pounds of muscle in 15 days. Take this power pack and lose all your fat in 30 days. Drink this tea and lose fat while you sleep and sit in the office. Do this 10-day cleanse to incinerate your body fat in record time.

Marketers realize that we're an emotional species. We want results immediately. We want to avoid struggle. We shy away from pain and seek comfort instead. We want the shortest route possible to our destination; who has time for the scenic route?

Basically, we're lazy.

All these personal characteristics play right into the hands of supplement companies and distributors, as they like to call themselves. This may sound as if I have a personal vendetta against supplement companies, which would be the furthest thing from the truth.

I do have an issue with messages and advertisements about the latest supplements or power packs promising results in a month's time. That is complete bullshit. That is manipulation. That is taking advantage of people who have good intentions but don't know any better. This isn't doing anyone a favor. This is a major reason why people develop negative associations with fitness and give up after failed attempts.

I like supplements when they're used in the right context for the correct reasons. Often, they aren't. Often, people are wasting their money and distancing themselves from the necessary steps it takes to succeed in fitness. These supplements promise people results. They promise people that if they buy their product, they'll essentially be skipping steps that other non-users have to go through.

In a nutshell, the majority of these sketchy supplement companies and distributors promise you that you can have your cake and eat it as well.

Unfortunately, fitness doesn't work that way. Fitness is tough, no other way to put it. If you want to look extraordinary and be remarkable, not just be an average Joe walking the streets, then you can't expect to take shortcuts and game the system.

Roll your sleeves up, prepare to get your hands dirty, and go to work by implementing the necessary habits and behaviors.

Supplements are for filling in deficiencies. Completing missing gaps. Serving as a Band-Aid on a small cut—not as a means to cover a flesh wound. That isn't going to suffice. Supplements are meant to supplement a sustainable diet that is missing a small piece to its puzzle. Hence the word supplement=support.

Relying on supplements programs you to solve your fitness woes with an instantaneous, short-term mindset. This is the same as buying bottle service and going on shopping sprees with a credit card when you have $10 in your checking account—no regard for the future, only concern for pleasure in the short-term.

Not only are you placing yourself further in the hole, but you're not learning valuable lessons that can only be learned through putting in the work each and every day.

Supplements don't improve your habits or teach you the proper skills needed for long-term success in fitness. They are not the answer to long-term transformations. No matter what you look to, short-term, instantaneous methods provide nothing but heartache, frustration, and empty pockets over the long haul.

Before you even think about buying supplements or the latest hydro, super, turbo whey protein, make sure your fundamentals are on point. Make sure your food choices are appropriate before thinking about a muscle-building protein stack. Using this stack as an extra boost to elicit greater muscle gains—not so good. Using it because you're having a hard time hitting your macros and reaching your caloric goals, food isn't easily accessible all day, or you're deficient in a mineral—now you're thinking clearly.

Doing a juice cleanse to lose fat when you haven't become consistent with exercising or with your eating habits—bad idea (you're avoiding the uncomfortableness of habit changing and seeking the easiest way out).

Before you spend a penny on supplements, make sure you spend that money on quality veggies and whole foods to eat. Supplements aren't the cure-all to your fitness woes nor can they help you avoid the necessary struggle, pain, and commitment that a fitness transformation requires.

Unless you have a deficiency of some sort in your diet or you naturally lack a particular nutrient or mineral, use that extra money for some new clothes after you morph into your new and improved physique.

Your mission, should you choose to accept: it

Before buying any supplements, make a checklist to ensure you have the basics covered first and are only purchasing based out of need or a deficiency.

Section IV

Lifestyle

Whether it's increasing time with friends, going on more dates, spending less time at work, or having more time for our hobbies, each of us has a particular lifestyle pictured inside our minds.

Lifestyle design takes top priority when it comes to making specific decisions and commitments. One of the most common excuses people use for not integrating a consistent fitness habit into their daily regimen is the claim that it takes away from their preferred lifestyle.

This is 100% true for those who approach their fitness in a restrictive and demanding mindset. Those who struggle with consistency in fitness approach a healthy lifestyle from a black-and-white perspective—it's either this way or it doesn't happen.

But you're not going to commit the same mistakes this time around. You're not going to let outdated dogmatic fitness philosophies engineer you into a lifestyle full of misery and resentment.

Constructing an optimal lifestyle starts with being aware of what you truly want—not what your friends, family, media, or anyone else determines for you. An optimal lifestyle flows seamlessly with your fitness habits. They complement each other, not compete against each other.

You have a life meant for adventure and experiences—however that looks to you. You have a unique dent to create in this universe, and your fitness needs to enhance these objectives, not cause a ruckus. Creating an optimal lifestyle that helps you thrive in fitness, excel in work, and live life on your own terms comes down to a focus on ten essential strategies that we're about to discuss.

Let's get to work on mastering these optimal lifestyle design strategies.

Strategy #21: Priorities...Priorities... Priorities

"Your actions speak so loudly, I cannot hear what you are saying."

—Ralph Waldo Emerson

"I need to start working out." "I need to start eating healthier." "I need to stop staying up so late."

"I need to stop wasting so much time on social media and increase my productivity." "I need to start reading more."

I need to this. I need to do that. I want to do this. I should do this. But this. But that. But, when I get some time.

Excuses. Blah Blah Blah.

Throughout our days, we all fall prey to blurting out something we want to do, but we just can't yet. Whether it's leaving the current dullness of our present lives behind in a pile of dust, traveling the world, leaving our jobs to chase down a dream, learning a language, learning how to dance, having a strong desire to level up our fitness—we let excuses prevent us from acting.

We have these desires, wants, and callings brewing inside of us, but no action takes place.

A disconnect between our wants, desires, and actions.

Beyond looking at excuses and using others as our scapegoats, it comes down to priorities. Plain and simple. If you keep telling yourself you should, that *should* needs to become your *must*.

If this fitness goal is important enough, you'll find a way to make it happen. Will it be tough? Absolutely. Will it be a linear and smooth-sailing path to success?

Not a puncher's chance in hell.

When you're going about your journey, you shouldn't expect seismic shifts. As we discussed earlier, when pursuing a fitness transformation or something outside your normal realm of comfort, baby steps, which feel and look insignificant, are vital.

Stating, "I would do this," or "I'll eventually get to..." isn't good enough.

This is the resistance controlling you. By waiting, you're procrastinating. Just start but don't place monumental pressure and expectations on yourself at the beginning.

For example, let's say you hate your job and want to chase down the digital nomad lifestyle. You wouldn't walk into the office the next day and quit without a plan for how you're going to make money and continue to pay your existing bills. What you would do instead is to continue to work, but use the time before and after to work on your freedom plan.

You want to pick up an exercise habit and lose fat, but you haven't worked out in months. You wouldn't dive headfirst into an intense five-day bodybuilding split. Instead, you'll make it a goal to simply get to the gym and exercise for 20 minutes two or three times a week.

It boils down to this...

You make time for what you really want. If the things you care about aren't being fit into your day, then you're prioritizing incorrectly. On the other hand, consider the possibility that you don't care as much as you think or proclaim to others about those particular goals.

It's okay if that's the case. Honesty is noble and commendable. If that isn't the case and you really do want those goals, then it's time to make necessary sacrifices. You claim work is crazy busy with no time for exercising; then wake up an hour earlier and head to the gym. Get off Facebook and Instagram, give up some of your favorite TV shows, and get to bed earlier so you can wake up and complete your workout.

Learn how to say no. It's one of the best words in your vocabulary. We often say yes out of obligation, guilt, and to pacify people's feelings. It's time for you to become a little selfish and put yourself—your body, mind, spirit, and emotions—first.

Does that feel selfish and too much for you?

Think of it this way. What good are you to the world if you're showing up each day a shell of what you could be? What good are you if you're showing up as half the person you could be?

By placing a priority on your health, you'll be able to create a bigger dent in the universe and truly become that shining star you were meant to become. The more intimate you become with your priorities, the greater your self-awareness will become about how you spend your time.

Your mission, should you choose to accept:

Take five minutes and think about something you want. Are you taking steps (big or small) each day to make this a reality?

If not, then why not? Answer this truthfully. Look at your daily routine and see what is replaceable with the actions needed to reach the goals you want. How could you make time for this goal? Make sure to line your priorities up with what you want out of life and fitness.

Strategy #22: The Dark Side of "Going with the Flow"

"If you talk about it, it's a dream, if you envision it, it's possible, but if you schedule it, it's real."

—Tony Robbins

Adrenaline is pumping through their veins, the new playlist is off the chain, and their gym attire is on point (maybe they'll find a date while they're at it).

This sound familiar?

This is the portrait of someone who has recently started down a fitness path.

Just like someone who has started a new job and is the best employee they can be for the first two weeks, they do everything right. Cleaning up the new diet they're on. Completing their recommended number of workouts throughout the week. Maintaining their blog weekly. Making those cool YouTube videos. Making that new squeeze a priority. The majority of us have zero problems being ultra-committed at the beginning. It's fun at the beginning, it's a novelty—like a jolt of lighting running through our veins, delivering us unfamiliar feelings.

"I've finally found the job of my dreams." "I'm on my way to being a prolific blogger and author."

"This relationship is so perfect and wonderful."

"I'm finally going to reach this weight loss goal and look fantastic in that sexy bikini."

Just when the fantasy of succeeding is flooding our thoughts, feelings, and dreams, Captain Reality once again makes his grand entrance.

It's week three of your program and things are going well until life throws you some curve balls with a couple fastballs mixed in. Unexpected work meetings, friends asking you out for social gatherings, and next thing you know, you've missed a couple sessions and you've gone off your nutrition plan. You planned to help your friend this afternoon and then workout; little did you know that it would take all day.

What happened?

The inability to follow through and fail proof your fitness habit is what happened.

Here's the lowdown.

At the beginning, creating a system and support team isn't necessary since you're in the adrenaline stage where it's exciting. This is your honeymoon phase. But, just as relationships lose their newness and cars lose that fresh smell, your fitness loses its luster.

Just as you schedule haircut appointments, when you'll be at work, and date nights, it's essential you schedule your gym time. When you "go with the flow and play it by ear," or "go when you have time," you're sending yourself down a dead end toward failure.

If it isn't on your schedule, it doesn't exist. Your gym time needs a designated timeslot on your schedule. Your gym slot is as important as your workday slot. It's important just like your haircut appointment. It's important just as that routine checkup at the doctor is. If it isn't on the schedule, you run the risk of letting other insignificant tasks sneakily sprout on the list and, next thing you know, you have no time for the gym.

By scheduling your workouts, you know when and where they will happen well in advance. Your fitness can't be left up to a roll of the dice. Your fitness needs to be concrete and operate like clockwork.

Your mission, should you choose to accept:

Do you have a designated time blocked off for the gym? If not, take some time and look over your schedule. Schedule your workout sessions for the week. This is one less thing to think about and one less thing to rely on willpower for (remember, willpower isn't to be trusted).

Once you schedule this time, stand firm and only break it for an emergency (a true emergency). Be militant about your times and priorities. Time is a resource that isn't renewable or replaceable.

Strategy #23: What Isn't Measured Doesn't Change

In my earlier days, my best friend and I were semi-ambitious college kids who had dreams of working for a trendy advertising agency, blurting out ideas every day and going to cool black-tie affairs at night.

Obviously, this scenario didn't pan out. I daydreamed through many of my business classes and subsequently ended up with a marketing degree. I do remember sitting through a logistics class when my instructor mentioned Peter Drucker ad nauseam and wrote his quote on the board: "What gets measured, gets managed."

Back in college, I was like "whatever" when I heard this. I had more important things on my mind such as "Is it workout time yet" or "Is it Thursday (thirsty Thursday anyone?)?"

Even though logistics is about as exciting as watching paint dry (sorry to some of my friends), this quote is gold when it comes to fitness. The concept makes sense—whatever you focus on improves. However, there's one potential problem that oftentimes bursts people's fitness bubbles—they're focused on the wrong things (or try to do too many things).

You can't improve everything at once.

Think about the lessons from *Moneyball*, starring Brad Pitt. For ages, baseball mangers scouted and analyzed talent in a particular way to make management decisions. *Moneyball* tells the story of two guys who are faced with unfavorable financial scenarios but still need to produce a competitive team. Instead of following the status quo, they end up analyzing talent through sabermetrics, which measures in-game activity. This unconventional method of scouting led the 2002 Oakland Athletics team to winning 20 games in a row (not too shabby).

Let's assume you want to lose fifteen pounds. You need to measure a few key factors such as waist measurements, body fat percentage, scale weight, and performance in the gym. You want all of these factors to improve; they all fit perfectly with the main goal of someone who wants to lose fifteen pounds.

Your actions and goals have to match up with your measurements. If you want to lose fifteen pounds, you know you need to eat healthier and strength train.

You'll break this down further by asking yourself:

1. Does my training and eating strategy align with my overall goal of fat loss?

2. Does this plan make sense? Is this plan sustainable?

3. If I do this training and diet plan, will I get the results that I want and how will I know? Will I use measurement tape biweekly as my barometer? Will I take progress pics every two to three weeks? Will I have a friend measure me? Will I get my body fat tested by a professional every four to seven weeks?

Your mission, should you choose to accept:

Think about how you will measure your progress. Pick out two to three methods and stick with them throughout the program.

Strategy #24: Become an Artist & Develop a Ritual to Catapult Yourself to Success

A ritual is a habit automatically triggered by a specific behavior that you perform. A ritual serves as a water hose and extinguishes your potential fires (i.e., procrastinations and various excuses).

American dancer and choreographer Twyla Tharp, author of *The Creative Habit: Learn It and Use It for Life*, used the same ritual to start her day and increase productivity.

She describes it this way, *"I begin each day of my life with a ritual: I wake up at 5:30 A.M., put on my workout clothes, my leg warmers, my sweatshirts, and my hat. I walk outside my Manhattan home, hail a taxi, and tell the driver to take me to the Pumping Iron Gym at 91st Street and First Avenue, where I work out for two hours.*

The ritual is not the stretching and weight training I put my body through each morning at the gym; the ritual is the cab. The moment I tell the driver where to go I have completed the ritual."

As Tharp explains, *"A ritual is a simple act, but doing it the same way each morning habitualizes it—it makes it repeatable, easy to do. It reduces the chance that I would skip it or do it differently. It is one more item in my arsenal of routines, and one less thing to think about."*

Establishing rituals isn't just for creatives; it also has value for the everyday person—the person who has to juggle many various daily duties along with trying to start a fitness habit. A fitness ritual isn't performing a set of squats or walking into the gym: it's the behavior that starts the entire process of going to the gym. The process of getting yourself to the gym is the overlooked aspect of mastering the habit of exercising.

Your success with rituals and fitness is determined by how sustainable the triggering mechanism is. Automating your habits leads to greater fat loss results, better quality of life, and less stress.

Warning: this isn't always easy.

If igniting a ritual to get you going were easy, there wouldn't be an obesity epidemic and diabetes wouldn't steadily be climbing the charts along with a slew of other health issues.

As Tharp explains, *"It's vital to establish some rituals—automatic but decisive patterns of behavior—at the beginning of the creative process, when you are most at peril of turning back, chickening out, giving up, or going the wrong way."*

Sound familiar?

It's difficult to get started with the exercise habit because many resistances are obnoxiously whispering, "Stop," and you're most likely feeling uncomfortable with loads of uncertainty.

But, just as creatives, musicians, and artists need a ritual to keep themselves aligned during their work sessions, it's vital you focus on developing an effective ritual to guide you along your exercise journey.

There will be days where you don't feel like working out, days where cooking healthy meals is the last thing on your mind, days where you feel tempted to fall back into old habits and stop at the drive-thru out of convenience, days where you want to grab a pseudo healthy meal at the grocery store that comes out of a box (never a good idea).

There will be days where taking those first few steps into version 2.0 feels daunting, impossible, and draining. However, realize these initial steps are damn hard, but that's why you have your ritual to back you up.

As Tharp explains, *"First steps are hard; it's no one's idea of fun to wake up in the dark every day and haul one's tired body to the gym. Like everyone, I have days when I wake up, stare at the ceiling, and ask myself, Gee, do I feel like working out today? But the quasi-religious power I attach to this ritual keeps me from rolling over and going back to sleep."*

A simple process for constructing a fitness ritual

At the beginning, your main objective is to get going, no matter how ugly, awkward, or uncertain it feels. Develop a simple plan and adjust on the fly. The less intricate the starting process, the likelier you're going to succeed this time around. Something is better than nothing. Starting is everything. Here's the "nuts 'n' bolts" method to igniting your ritual.

1. Start small and keep your expectations within reason

The worst thing you can do when starting a fitness journey is to bombard yourself with a multitude of steps and intricate processes to activate your habit. Avoid the temptation of attaching an expected result to these early attempts.

At the beginning, you're throwing a bunch of darts against the board and seeing what sticks. These steps should almost feel effortless. Be easy on yourself about slip-ups. Decide where you currently stand with your fitness and nutritional habits. Be realistic and keep your expectations low—early and small wins are your ally. Run away from the all-or-none mentality and instead think 1% daily improvement.

2. Develop a process for your desired behavior

The tougher the barrier of entry, the less likely you are to stick with it for the long term. Make the process of entry into your ritual simple and concise by limiting the process to three to four steps for activation.

3. Know your signal to trigger your ritual

When does the ritual begin? What's the ignition to starting your engine?

In football terms, your ritual is the snap count. The entire offense has to be in harmony. From the lineman to the receivers, everyone has to know the snap count or a penalty occurs and the ref throws a flag.

For Twyla, the ritual was the cab itself—telling the driver where to go. For me, I set my timer, have a bottle of water, cup of coffee, & hit play on my Bossa Nova, neo-soul, or Marvin Gaye playlist depending on my mood—now I automatically understand it's time to write and perform my other work tasks.

A ritual for waking up in the morning would be the ringing of your alarm clock.

4. Don't be afraid to experiment with different flavors until you blend the magic brew

Have fun with the process. There'll be bumps along the road at the beginning when establishing a ritual. You'll only find the perfect steps by doing and seeing what works and what doesn't. Test, assess, and test some more.

Here's an example to get your ideas flowing for developing an exercise ritual:

Working out– The best way to set up an exercise ritual is to place it around the time with the least amount of resistances. Try setting up a fitness ritual first thing in the morning before any work related material or emails receive attention.

Alternatively, pack your gym clothes and exercise after work or during your lunch break (don't tell yourself you'll go home first and then go back). If you're lifting in the afternoon or evening, place your gym time on your schedule so nothing sneaks its way onto that specific time slot.

Your mission, should you choose to accept:

Start a ritual this week. Analyze your schedule and think of a sequence of events that could help you shift the habit of exercise closer to being automatic.

Strategy #25: Identify the Potential Villains in Your Life

We all have weaknesses. We all have specific environments where our fitness behaviors land in the dumpster. The most dedicated fitness soldier couldn't survive some of these temptations.

Having weaknesses and temptations doesn't make you less of a person. It means you're a human.

We all have particular environments and people that neutralize our strength, cripple our focus, and yank control away from us. These danger zones and villains are where our greatest battles occur.

Superman has Lex Luther. Captain America has Red Skull. Black Panther has Ulysses Klaw. Fantastic Four has Doctor Doom. Spider-Man has Green Goblin. Batman has the Joker. Flash has the Reverse Flash.

We everyday intelligent, creative, ambitious, and remarkable individuals have plenty of villains in our lives just as these superheroes do.

All villains aren't psychotic or outwardly evil—some are unintentionally a danger to our fitness goals. Certain villains only morph into villains due to their specific circumstances and environments. The most dangerous kinds of villains unintentionally become a detriment to our fitness goals. They're the people who are often the closest to us.

We've seen villains materialize from best friends, neighbors, coworkers, significant others, family members, mentors, and the media. You don't have to eliminate all your fitness villains, but you must take control and use the power of awareness to harness your foe.

Take the first step toward controlling the villains along your fitness journey by asking, "What temptations in my day-to-day life have the possibility of derailing my fitness goals?"

Is it your closest friends who have poor eating habits, thus making you feel guilty for attempting to practice healthier eating habits? Is it your stressful, negative, and annoying coworkers who make you more susceptible to snacking throughout the day? Is it your family who guilts you into eating their traditionally home-cooked meals, even if it goes against your dietary goals and beliefs? Is it pressure from a significant other to eat their food? Are they guilting you into having a couple obligatory drinks nightly?

Does your environment lack healthy eating alternatives come lunchtime? Is it not having the right support system around you to encourage positive habits toward reaching your goals?

Whatever the issue, it's essential you take the time to figure out the danger zones of your life and the villains who pose a threat to building the body you want.

Ask yourself, "What am I going to do in order to not let these daily temptations sabotage me and my fitness goals?"

Is it explaining boundaries to family? Removing the guilt for not drinking with friends? Packing your lunch so there's no question what you're going to eat and no temptation to blame your surroundings for poor food decisions?

Whatever it is, it's essential you develop a solution that fits your lifestyle like Velcro.

Your mission, should you choose to accept:

Acknowledge your villains. Embrace the challenges they pose and the potential power they have. Establish a strategy of how you'll go about defeating your villains whenever they decide to create a ruckus.

Strategy #26: Become an Avenger & Leverage the Power of Support & Accountability

From Thor to Iron Man to Captain America to the Incredible Hulk to Black Widow to Scarlet Witch to Hawkeye—the Avengers are invincible from a surface perspective.

But you can't always judge a book by its cover or take everything at face value. Each of the Avengers faces their fair share of adventures and dangerous foes as a solo act, but they always come out victorious.

So why would they need help from each other?

Simple.

Whether a superhero or trained assassin, one person can only do so much. One person can only handle so many burdens before becoming overwhelmed. One person can only carry so much on their shoulders before they tip over. Sometimes, the battle that lies ahead requires a team effort due to the power of the resistances at hand (e.g., Ultron or the Chitauri army).

At the beginning of their partnership, the Avengers are reluctant—too stubborn to trust each other and ask for help. They're operating from an ego standpoint, instead of acting logically and doing whatever is required to accomplish the mission. Eventually, they receive their call to action and realize that saving the world can't be accomplished through their solo efforts and powers. If they are to save the world, it will take them cooperating as a unit and utilizing each other's unique skill sets.

Fitness presents the same predicament as superheroes trying to save the world.

For years, I struggled with reaching out for help and asking others to help me stay accountable. At the beginning of my exercise journey, I attempted highly technical exercises, even though I wasn't 100% proficient or confident in them (luckily no serious injuries happened). My ego prevented me from asking the person beside me doing them because I figure it would make me less of a man. Sounds crazy, but men especially have huge egos.

No matter the venture or activity in life, you can't succeed alone.

You can't succeed in business without networking. A relationship isn't a success with only one out of two participants. Michael Jordan didn't win six championships by himself. Someone has to call the plays to make the players look good. Hit records aren't a solo endeavor. You get the drift...

You can't succeed in fitness alone.

If superheroes can't save the world by themselves, why would you expect yourself to conquer fitness without support and accountability?

We tend to underestimate the amount of effort required—physically, emotionally, and mentally—to achieve what we aspire to in life.

From figuring out what kind of training program to implement to figuring out how to perform those exercises correctly, from committing to attending the gym on a regular basis to eating the correct macros to fuel your daily energy and workout levels—the list is endless.

Combine these gym factors with your everyday responsibilities of work, family significant others, and other miscellaneous responsibilities, and your plate is quickly overloading and starting to fall onto the floor. However, before your plate overfills with responsibilities and you start pulling your hair out, or, even worse, give up due to feeling overwhelmed...

Leverage the power of people and seek out support and accountability.

Each member of the Avengers brings a unique power to the group. Scout and recruit family, friends, coworkers, and whoever else can specifically complement your needs. Some people are natural motivators, while others are tacticians with exercise programming, and others are nutritional wizards.

I'm a fitness professional with over a decade's worth of experience, and even I at times have difficulty juggling my workouts with writing, attempting to show some semblance of coordination on the dance floor, and coaching clients.

Knowing this, I leveraged the power of the people and recruited one of my more fiery friends to light a fire under my ass to help me become consistent again with fitness. As much as we like to think we're invincible and can handle loads and loads of stress and responsibilities, we're lying to ourselves.

Without accountability, you're operating with a broken system. Accountability and support are the secret weapons that many successful artists, high-functioning executives, and fitness professionals use to stay focused and survive those days when adrenaline and magical motivational dust doesn't show up.

Here are six options to bring accountability & support into your life

1. Visual evidence – Taking biweekly measurements of key areas along with pictures is an excellent way to keep yourself accountable. We're visual creatures and what better way to keep ourselves focused than a picture of us standing with little clothing on to remind of us of the work we want to accomplish over the next couple of months (the camera doesn't lie).

2. Keep up with your workouts and food intake – While tracking your food intake for the rest of your life is a silly idea, at the beginning, it's a good idea to track your food to understand just what and how much you're eating on a daily basis.

How do you know your progress in the gym if you don't keep up with what you're doing? Keeping up with your workouts allows you to remain focused in the gym and not veer off with pointless exercises and waste time.

3. Let the world know your goals (or at least a few trusted sources) – Not everyone needs to know your business, but keep a couple people in the loop about what you're trying to accomplish. We all could use someone to call us out on our BS when we're slacking.

4. Find a workout partner (a serious one) – A best friend who is real chatty isn't going to cut it. If you don't have another option, establish some rules beforehand. Keep a timer and agree to stick to the prescribed rest periods.

5. Take photos of your food – No, this isn't just to post on Instagram (we already know you're a self-professed foodie). These pictures are designed to bring awareness into your decision making when eating. It's a great visual representation of what you actually eat. It's one thing to write it down, but to actually see what you're eating creates a stronger input in your mind.

Taking pictures of food and then having to share it will make you think twice about eating foods that aren't conducive toward your fitness goals.

6. Put some skin in the game – My favorite. This one is about being bold and confident in your ability to do what you say you're going to do.

Giving lip service is one thing, but often it's nothing more than hot air and oxygen being released (maybe bad breath, as well). There isn't a stronger and more effective way than making a commitment contract or putting some money on the line. Write a contract up with your stated goals and lay out the rewards and consequences of achieving versus not achieving. Include a couple friends and this method is almost fail proof due to competition.

Warning: an effective contract isn't primarily focused on measuring pounds. Make the stipulations focused on taking the correct actions. Be process/system oriented, not goal/result oriented—you can control the actions of the process, not the end-result (from a timeframe standpoint).

Your mission, should you choose to accept:

Think about an area of fitness in which you're currently struggling. Then, think about your network and reach out to someone who you think could help you on your specific issue. After finding someone, choose one or two of the six options above to bring some accountability into your fitness life.

Strategy #27: Break Down Your Day into Quarters

"What you do every day matters more than what you do once in a while."

—Gretchen Rubin

At one point in my fitness journey, there were days where I went on a Red Vines binge or accidentally ate a couple slices of pizza in the early afternoon. Other days, I binged on a few too many desserts at lunch with friends.

This threw off my total macros for the day—now my calories weren't going to be exactly what I intended them to be. Afterwards, I felt like a failure and labeled the day as a waste since I'd screwed up my macros. What's the point of eating correctly the rest of the day if I've already blown my macros and eaten foods that weren't included in my daily nutrition plan?

This was my mindset and approach with food. One mistake during the day and it caused me to go into a tailspin. Since I'd already ruined my day "eating the wrong foods," I gave myself a dietary get-out-of-jail-free card and declared that current day a free-for-all, promising myself that I'd jump back onto the dietary wagon starting tomorrow (a dangerous game to play).

I frequently meet people who approach their nutrition with the mindset that if you eat off your plan earlier in the day, then the day is a waste and deserves a mulligan.

Since the day is a mulligan, you might as well eat additional foods that aren't conducive to your physique goals. This makes sense to them because they're "emptying their system of the bad food cravings." Come tomorrow, it's time to eat clean and train dirty. They're going to be spot on with their nutrition and training habits.

Sure, tell yourself that. I've resided in the land of denial for extensive periods playing this game. Not only is this game dangerous because it forces you to seek perfection (a fairy tale), but it also teaches you to treat nutrition with an all-or-none mentality.

Nutrition isn't an all-or-none activity. One mistake or turn off the desired course of travel doesn't mean you can't salvage the day.

Missing an entry onto the freeway doesn't mean you can't merge later on down the road. If you're playing poorly the entire first half, that doesn't mean you can't rebound in the second half and turn the game around.

You made some mistakes earlier in the day, or had a meal or two that threw your daily macros off. That doesn't mean you've failed the day or yourself. What it means is that you're a human filled with emotions, not a machine lacking a pulse and hormones.

Instead of playing with fire and using this all-or-none mentality, keep the big picture in mind.

Your new fitness game plan: Break your day down into quarters

Gretchen Rubin, author of *Better than Before* states, *"Instead of feeling that you've blown the day and thinking, I'll get back on track tomorrow, try thinking of each day as a set of four quarters: morning, midday, afternoon, evening. If you blow one quarter, you get back on track for the next quarter. Fail small, not big."*

Occasionally veering off your course isn't going to swing the pendulum in the wrong direction if you usually eat for your desired body. A couple unexpected happy hour drinks or dessert over lunch won't make a dent or even a scratch with your physique goals if you're making the right decisions over the course of each day.

If you're dialed in 90% of the time, pay no attention to the other 10% when life happens or you just want to enjoy yourself.

There's much more to this thing we call life than abiding by the "Instagram bro & broette code" where it's balls to the walls every day (every day is beastmode), and where there are countless food prep pictures, fitspo inspiration quotes, shirtless pictures with some empty motivational quote below, or any other fitness mumbo-jumbo.

Whoa. I didn't mean to start preaching. Sometimes you catch the spirit. Back to our normal program.

Stay present and maintain the big perspective of your situation. As soon as you catch yourself off course, the key is to get back aboard the dietary wagon as soon as possible to prevent old habits from sneaking back into your life.

Your mission, should you choose to accept:

Think of your day as quarters. Which one do you struggle with? Think about some changes that you can make to turn that quarter into a positive. Once you determine the quarter that you want to focus on, implement one action toward this quarter.

Strategy #28: Morph Your Macro Goals into Micro Goals

"Great things are done by a series of small things brought together."

—Vincent van Gogh

Ambition is one of our greatest assets when it comes to creating change within our lives. However, on the opposite end of the spectrum, ambition has the ability to become our worst enemy. Ambition possesses the ability to cloud our judgement and make us impatient with our goals.

With sexy, half-clothed, flawless bodies spamming our Instagram and Facebook newsfeeds, our patience shortens and emotions start to overtake us.

We want our goals and we want them now. Marketers juggle our emotions with 30-day physique transformation stories. The news feeds us overnight success stories. Social media makes us feel as if everyone is in shape besides ourselves. But those overnight transformations are anything but an overnight success story. Those overnight success stories can be months or even years in the making. Comparing ourselves to those we see across various news and social media outlets is unfair and never leaves us in a winning situation.

Never compare your first draft to someone else's final draft. Never compare your behind-the-scenes with someone else's feature film. Never compare your internal world with someone else's curated external world.

No one goes from zero to hero in one day. No one morphs into Arnold or a Sports Illustrated model in 21 days. Transformations take time. I didn't go from a 165-pound kid into a 200-pound adult in one swift flick of the wrist.

By obsessing over the big (macro) goal, you're potentially setting yourself up for doubt, pessimism, and feelings of inferiority. Obsessing over the big goal often leads one to looking ahead well into the future, but forgetting to appreciate the present moment and the progress accomplished on a daily basis.

Let's look at an example.

Janice wants to lose 25 pounds. Losing this amount of weight in a safe and sustainable way that is beneficial both internally and externally takes time (no way around this). The long journey ahead may at times feel never-ending, especially in the middle stages, as she seems to be in no man's land (i.e., a place where progress is hard to define and assess).

In addition, Janice is a beginner with brief exposure to fitness and hasn't experienced much success with fitness in her past. In addition to most likely being impatient and having unrealistic expectations (thanks to her external influences), she's battling past demons and self-doubt (which is a beast itself).

Twenty-five pounds is a big deal. This amount is going to take months. Therefore, it's crucial that Janice builds momentum to keep moving toward her transformation. As we learned earlier, momentum is crucial to sticking with a lifestyle change.

The best solution for Janice is to set up a few micro goals. Instead of celebrating and feeling justified only once she reaches 25 pounds, she should set smaller benchmarks that are attainable in shorter periods. These smaller benchmarks add gasoline to the fire and keep her marching toward her big goal while feeling confident about herself in the present moment.

No one wants to keep performing an activity if they never see or feel any benefits stemming from it. We all like to feel like winners, hence the power of micro goals in producing small wins. An initial milestone for Janice could be losing her initial five pounds.

Losing 5 pounds sounds a hell of a lot easier than losing 25 pounds. The mind is a delicate entity, and we must treat it that way. Give yourself the advantage by heading into your fitness transformation with the correct mindset. Only worry about losing those initial 5 pounds and nothing else. Five comes before 25. Ten comes before 25. Being able to celebrate milestones every few weeks is better than waiting to give yourself permission to celebrate four to six months down the road.

Set up small victories. If five sounds daunting or if you're a total beginner, initially nervous, or you've experienced past failures with fitness, start with losing three pounds and build from that.

Life doesn't need to be put on hold until you reach your target number. You deserve and need to celebrate the small victories as well. Rome wasn't built in a day. Lego pieces aren't built in one connection. Storybook romances won't happen overnight and neither will fat loss. But that doesn't mean we can't celebrate each and every pound along the way.

Your mission, should you choose to accept:

Once you have your fat loss goal or whatever your fitness goal is, take your big end goal and break it down into small chunks. Once you hit each of those small goals, treat yourself to a small celebration (don't be lazy and just binge on junk food; get creative).

Strategy #29: Everlasting Love & the Power of Sleep

We've all been there at one point in our lives.

It's an overwhelming feeling. One that at times makes you do stupid things. One that causes you to blurt out illogical thoughts fueled by passion. One that keeps you awake at night with anticipation and visions of what life's going to be like in the future. Sometimes you forget to eat. Sometimes you have butterflies in your stomach and are at a loss for words.

What am I talking about?

I'm talking about L-O-V-E—the kind that Al Green described back in 1975.

We've all been head over heels about that special someone. Maybe it was an enchanting summer fling, a timeless romance abroad, an innocent Internet conversation that morphed into a new-age Tom Hanks & Meg Ryan romantic comedy, or a chance encounter at the art gallery that morphed into something magical.

Each of those scenarios has a common thread—passion was bountiful. When you're in love, the object of your affections is put on a pedestal and treated with the utmost respect.

Whether you're a fitness veteran or a complete newbie learning the ropes of fitness, one thing that you need to remember is that sleep needs to be placed on a pedestal.

We live in a world where we're encouraged to party like a rock star, keep going till the sun comes up, work until we drop. If you're tired and feel like sleeping, don't be a pansy and quit—drink this five-hour energy drink and get back to hustling. We live in a culture where we brag about grinding and hustling 24/7. Unfortunately, this "hustling" and "going beastmode" epidemic isn't just limited to the business world.

Our fitness is just as infected. We're encouraged to train balls to the wall and leave nothing in the tank. More cardio. More workouts. More,

more, more—will it ever be enough? After all, you can sleep when you die.

This logic is utter rubbish.

Just as the love of your life is a priority that you treat with respect, your sleep deserves the same.

Have a seat at the fitness orchestra

Imagine that you're dressed fancifully and are listening to the orchestra at the symphony hall. Beautiful, melodic music is flowing in the hallways. A vast array of instruments is wooing the audience, each playing a different part for that particular composition.

When these sounds come together, perfection is witnessed (or harmony, if you're literal). Just as an orchestra needs all its musicians to be on their A game to achieve the highest level of performance, our bodies have a slew of hormones that must work together harmoniously to succeed in the mission of fat loss.

Each hormone (i.e., each instrument) has a specific role to play and when their powers are combined (just like in Captain Planet) with the appropriate amount of sleep, you're supplying a key cornerstone toward building the body you want.

A brief blurb on the dark side of no sleep

Sleep deprivation can cause a ruckus, impacting your body and your psyche. A couple of hormones that play a crucial role in sleep are listed below, along with how a lack of sleep affects them.

Insulin – In addition to making you cranky, sleep deprivation affects the way your body responds to insulin. Your insulin sensitivity starts to decrease, thus causing your body to not use insulin properly. Over time this leads to potential weight gain.

Leptin and Ghrelin – Lack of sleep reduces leptin and elevates your ghrelin levels, thus increasing appetite, which explains erratic food behaviors throughout your days.

Cortisol – Known as our stress hormone. While stress is a natural occurrence and is beneficial at times, sleep deprivation will cause this hormone to spike beyond normal levels.

This in turn slows our fat loss and increases potential weight gain over time because cortisol inhibits insulin from transporting glucose into our cells. Not to get too sciencey, but this means there's lots of glucose floating around in our bloodstreams. Glucose that isn't transported to our livers and muscle and stored as glycogen is most likely taking a trip to your fat cells.

Human growth hormone – Helps repair the body, strengthen bones, boost collagen production (leading to fewer wrinkles), and increase muscle mass. Skimping on sleep will release more cortisol, thus causing the body to release less growth hormone.

Sleep deprivation causes us to have less focus and concentration throughout the day as well as decreased working memory. If it comes down to sleep or an extra workout, sleep wins 100% of the time. Without sleep, progress is unlikely. Let me repeat, without sleep, you won't see progress and you'll be left in frustration.

Your mission, should you choose to accept:

Make sleep a "no ifs, ands, or buts" priority. Settle for no less than seven hours (within all your power). If you're chronically below this number, start gradually getting closer to seven by going to sleep 30 minutes earlier for a few days and gradually pushing up your bedtime until your goal number is reached.

Strategy #30: Everyone Needs Constraints

It's easy to complain that we have too little time, a lack of skills, not enough money, subpar looks, or a lack of resources—we just have too many constraints holding us back.

In some instances, it's true, these constraints are holding us back. In most cases though, these constraints are a positive waiting to be un-wrapped. Constraints in our daily lives force us to make decisions and sac-rifices, rise to the occasion, and harness our talents.

Constraints spark remarkability, creativity, and new skills and help us accomplish fitness goals. Constraints have changed my life. They've forced me to leave my comfort zone, get over the fear of perfection, and let go of the fear of rejection.

One of the best examples of the positive power of constraints comes from Dr. Seuss and the bet he was involved in. Someone placed a bet with him that he couldn't write a children's book using only 50 different words. That book became *Green Eggs and Ham*. He obviously succeeded.

Constraints are your best friend because they force you to show up and deliver, regardless of your situation, thus preventing you from pro-crastinating and only doing the work when "you feel like it."

Utilizing the power of constraints enabled me to take my writing, productivity, and life to another level by establishing a commitment and operating with consistent regularity.

I wanted to write consistently. I started with 250 words per day, then 500, then 1000. I knew that making a writing commitment would be uncomfortable. Some days I don't feel like writing. The weather is nice, beautiful girls keep walking by at the coffee shop, my room is dirty, I want some ice cream, or any other random excuse that pops up—anything to let me off the hook from writing.

While traveling, visiting friends, or sitting in an airport, I made sure to stick to this commitment, come hell or high water. Without establishing a commitment (schedule/constraint), I wouldn't have hit my goals. You wouldn't be reading this book and I would still be staring at the girls through the window (most likely not talking; I'm kinda shy), and twiddling my thumbs.

These constraints we put on ourselves turns us pro, as Steven Pressfield says, and it eliminates the option of procrastination. Constraints make you have a schedule, which forces you to do something, even if it isn't perfect.

Sound familiar?

Fitness operates under the same umbrella. At the beginning, it's tough, uncomfortable, and difficult. You're worried about how you look, whether you're in the right program, on the right diet, following the right approach. You wonder if you will succeed. There are thousands of thoughts and feelings circulating inside that crazy and beautiful brain of yours.

And that's 100% ok.

This feeling of not enough time, not enough knowledge, not being good enough, or whatever you feel you don't have enough of isn't an excuse not to show up and do the work.

There's a saying in the creative community that professionals show up regardless of whether the muse is with them, regardless of whether they feel inspired or not, while amateurs wait for inspiration.

Professionals get work done. Professionals achieve their fitness transformations. Professionals finish their books. Professionals get their promotions. Professionals get the girls. Professionals show up. Professionals take action.

Amateurs talk a good game. Amateurs share inspiring pictures through social media while doing nothing else. Amateurs blame their fitness woes on external factors. Amateurs have incomplete books. Amateurs daydream 24/7. Amateurs rely on creepy pick-up artist tactics. Amateurs are pretenders.

Which are you? Which will you be? Will you take action?

Got 30 minutes to work out? Great, that's plenty of time, get to work. Got 15 minutes to work out? Great, make it a damn good 15 minutes. We all have constraints and various roadblocks in our lives. Make the best of whatever time, resources, money, or knowledge you have and get to work. Remarkability doesn't settle for excuses.

The stoics say, "While we can't control the environment and actions around us, we can choose how we will respond to those situations."

Build your fitness skills and embrace your constraints by…

1. **Deciding on the goal you want to reach.**

2. **Thinking about the constraints around this particular goal. Is it perceived lack of time, resources, or environment? –** Whatever it is, recognize it and own it. If it's time, set a workout schedule that forces you to show up. Plan it out to avoid excuses.

3. **Just showing up –** At the beginning, it's rough and you might suck, but that's okay and unavoidable. There's beauty in the beginning when you're developing your skills.

Fitness is a skill just like painting and music. Picasso wasn't Picasso on day one. Henri Matisse wasn't Henri Matisse on day one. Prince wasn't Prince on day one. Ray Charles wasn't Ray Charles on day one.

Show up and play the game. Put your coins in and step up to the joystick. Get your reps in. Start your 10,000 hours of mastery, as Malcolm Gladwell states.

Your mission, should you choose to accept:

Identify at least one constraint in your life and turn this potential obstacle into a strength by determining a strategy for it and integrating it into your lifestyle.

Section V

Training

"Physical fitness is not only one of the most important keys to a healthy body, it is the basis of dynamic and creative intellectual activity."

—John F. Kennedy

Perhaps you expected the discussion of training to come first? Contrary to popular opinion, the actual workout itself is the least important pillar we've discussed. As a person who has experimented with many types of training programs, I can guarantee you with 100% certainty that the type of training program you do isn't close to being one of the most important decisions you make toward mastery of your fitness.

What good does a training program accomplish if your mindset isn't aligned with your goals at hand? The best training program in the world won't help you if your diet isn't a priority and isn't given the proper attention it deserves. What good is a training program that ultimately imprisons you in a lifestyle that isn't to your liking and strips away your identity?

Training gets in where it fits in. There are many different paths to the top of the mountain; it all depends on how you want to go about climbing it. Training goes beyond merely showing up to do a workout. Going to the gym for 45 minutes isn't just what a good training lifestyle is about.

A good training lifestyle is similar to how Steve Jobs describes design: *"Design is not just what it looks like and feels like. Design is how it works."*

A solid training lifestyle flows seamlessly from your mindset, thrives off your positive nutrition habits, emotionally catapults you to greatness in your specific line of work, and meshes flawlessly with your desired lifestyle.

Without further ado, let's discuss the ten essential training strategies toward mastery of one's fitness.

Strategy #31: Strength Training Is Your Foundation

Just as you can't build a house without a foundation, learn how to salsa dance without an understanding of the basic steps, become an opera singer without an understanding of vocal control, or become the next Coltrane without control of your breath, you can't reach a high level of fitness without strength training.

Strength training has many different associations and identities.

Some circles may associate strength training with bros and broettes unapologetically embracing vanity while curling in front of the mirror. Some may associate strength training with the obnoxious behaviors that take place on Instagram (just check some fitness related hashtags if you need an introduction). Some circles may still view strength training as something for the elite who want excessive muscles, not something for the casual guy or gal who just wants to shape up and lose a couple inches. Lastly and most unfortunate, many people are intimidated by the thought of strength training.

I understand where each of these impressions stems from. Before reframing my mindset, I felt that strength training was 100% focused on aesthetics and to hell with the other benefits.

Before moving on, I must state this—strength training is for everyone, not just for the elite, meatheads, bros, the guy who's severely into himself, or any other character that may be circulating inside your mind. Strength training may look and mean different things to each of us, but don't dismiss your meaning because it's not a popular/mainstream interpretation.

Damn. Sorry, I caught the spirit again.

While strength training benefits our appearance, the benefits extend beyond this. Strength training provides us the opportunity to educate and train our body and mind simultaneously. In addition to helping fight off certain diseases, strength training teaches us the power of commitment and consistency.

Strength training needs to be a nonnegotiable part of our lives. We go to the doctor for checkups, we never miss an episode of *Game of Thrones* (unless you've haven't seen an episode, like me), some of us never miss an episode of reality TV (I'm sorry for your addictions), we make a priority to watch college football religiously...why not make strength training a priority?

However, let's first create a mini-bio for what strength training encompasses.

The proper way to describe strength training

When you think of strength training, think of it as a form of exercise that's used to strengthen your mind as well as your musculoskeletal system.

Wait...What did you just say?

Your musculoskeletal system is comprised of bones, muscles, cartilage, tendons, ligaments, joints, and connective tissues that help bind your tissues and organs together. Our musculoskeletal system provides support, stability, movement, and form to our bodies.

Strength training/resistance training/weight lifting, or whatever other fanciful name you would like to use, builds our relative and absolute strength, our endurance, and the size of our muscles, and improves our "tone."

The vast benefits of strength training

Some people strength train so they can take beach photos and or because they think their chances of getting laid will increase with this activity. But strength training contains a slew of other benefits to encourage you to start immediately (if you haven't already).

You decrease your chances of osteoporosis – Osteoporosis is a condition where your bones break down and become weaker. Women are twice as likely as men to suffer from this condition, which makes strength training that much more beneficial. Resistance training has proven beneficial to improving bone density, which lowers your chances for osteoporosis.

You improve stability and balance – No, I'm not talking about squatting on a bosu ball or any other device (this isn't the circus). Instead, you're focusing on exercises such as planks, compound exercises, and single leg work such as lunges, Bulgarian split squats (my fav), and single leg RDLs that will improve your day-to-day functioning.

Everyday activities are improved – Walking with your kids, walking with a date in the park (underrated), going for a jog, and picking up boxes around the house get easier as you start to strength train and build up your body.

Low back pain vanishes like a thief in the middle of the night due to strengthening your hamstrings and glutes. Most of the time when you hear peers and coworkers complaining of back pain, it's due to weak hamstrings and sleepy glutes (we sit way too much).

Body composition changes for the better – Relying on "long duration cardio" in the form of running on the treadmill, peddling away on a stationary bike, climbing the stairway to heaven on the StairMaster, or using the elliptical will result in some weight loss (because diet is the domino factor no matter what).

The type of weight loss occurring without strength training is one where you're just a smaller version of yourself, but not necessarily an improved version from a physical aesthetics perspective. Since resistance training isn't being implemented, you're not undergoing force adaptations within the body.

What do I mean?

This type of weight loss won't remove man boobs, or a skinny fat appearance if that's your goal. Implementing resistance training into your regimen positively alters your appearance due to increased muscle and improved shape (tone).

It sounds better to lose five pounds of fat and gain five pounds of muscle than to only lose five pounds. You'll weigh the same but your body fat has decreased while lean body weight has increased. Think fat loss, not weight loss.

General health – Strength training causes a decrease in stress, blood pressure, heart rate, cholesterol levels, type 2 diabetes, and helps slow down the aging process (can we say forever young?). Expect increases in sleep quality, libido, energy levels, insulin sensitivity, and cardiovascular endurance, and a reduced incidence of injury.

Mental well-being – This is by far the most important benefit of lifting weights (for me personally). Depression and anxiety lowers in individuals who engage in strength training. Studies have indicated that resistance training helps improve memory, cognition, and self-esteem.

Displaying an eye-catching physique is a great goal, but having self-confidence and a positive self-image should be at the top of your priority list as you venture through this thing we call life and fitness.

Your mission, should you choose to accept:

Commit to attempting strength training if you haven't already. Lay out the top three reasons strength training will benefit you personally that don't involve getting laid or looking hot in a bikini (those are too obvious). Knowing your reasons is your ammunition for continuing when you might not feel like it or feel scared.

Don't overwhelm yourself at the beginning. Commit to two to three days for as little as 15-20 minutes if this type of activity is new.

Strategy #32: Compound Exercises are the Bread & Butter of Your Operation

Bulging biceps. Tight and toned stomach. Lean and lovely legs. Perky glutes.

The majority of us, as we're initially beginning to work out, tend to pinpoint certain areas of our body to target. Our bodies are a dart board, and we're aiming for the bullseye (our specific target body part). Whether it's tightening our thighs, trimming stomach fat, or trying to make our chest and biceps standout for the upcoming beach season, we approach our training methodologies from an isolation mindset.

Many of us have numerous day-to-day responsibilities and hobbies, thus making our time that more precious. Time is sacred and isn't renewable, therefore efficiency is priority. This makes the isolation mentality highly ineffective and wasteful (especially for beginners).

It is a myth that you can reduce a particular area by performing isolation exercises such as bicep curls, tricep kickbacks, leg extensions, hip abductors, and many others.

You can perform sit-ups to your heart's content or curl until your arms no longer rise, but your belly fat and any dangling arm fat won't necessarily vanish. Isolation exercises provide additional volume to help the muscularity of a particular muscle, but that is a moot point if there are still layers of fat on top of that particular area. Isolation exercises alone won't incinerate fat from any particular area.

Allow me to introduce you to compound exercises (where efficiency meets effectiveness)

Compound exercises are multi-jointed movements that work one or more muscle groups per movement. Compound exercises such as squats, deadlifts, hip thrust, Bulgarian split squats, overhead presses, bench presses, chin-ups, and pull-ups provide more bang for the buck per movement than isolation exercises.

Compound movements provide neural, hormonal, and cellular responses within the body, which helps you maintain lean body mass (i.e., keeping your muscles while losing fat) and create a greater caloric expenditure within the body for each workout (i.e., burning more calories). Due to the efficient nature of implementing compound exercises within each workout, you're able to recruit a higher number of motor units within the body, which elicits muscle growth.

Compound exercises allow you to build coordination and, most important, they save you vast amounts of time in the gym compared to having a routine full of isolation movements. Think quality, not quantity when it comes to time.

Being a busy professional, creative, artist, or someone new to fitness, it's imperative that you cement a solid foundation and focus on the big wins.

Think about the Pareto principle used in business: 80% of your sales (i.e., results) come from 20% of the entire operation (i.e., customers). In fitness, 20% of your strength training (compound movements) will give you 80% of your results. Once again, think quality, not quantity (just remember this for every facet of your life).

Creating a routine with the majority comprising compound movements slashes your time and triples your results per session (therefore providing more time for experiencing life).

Before you start worrying about targeting a specific body part, focus on creating an overall solid training base. With every workout, I recommend you start with a compound movement and, maybe at the end, throw some isolation exercises into the mix.

Your mission, should you choose to accept:

Look over your current workout program and make sure each training session begins with a compound movement. Remember to make the majority of your exercises compound movements. Fewer exercises per session, but exercises that are more effective, is the model of excellence.

Strategy #33: Train for Strength at the Beginning (And Leave Everything Else by the Wayside)

At the beginning of the fitness journey, you're visualizing how you'll look and feel filling out a T-shirt. You're visualizing how stunning you'll look in that stylish bikini. You visualize having a set of head-turning glutes as you walk down the street. You're anticipating what it is going to feel like to be the inspiration for others when they get ready to make their transformation.

You're anticipating proving the doubters and haters wrong. You may also be anticipating how it's going to feel to make your exes and old prospects jealous (it's okay to admit this). Most important, you're anticipating the confidence that a fitness transformation will bring from an emotional, physical, spiritual, and mental standpoint.

This over-eagerness can lead you to perform a gazillion sets of kickbacks, machine presses, and leg extensions. While those exercises are valuable depending on the goal and trainee, at the beginning, those exercises won't properly serve you.

Strength and only strength is your focus before getting fancy with other training metrics.

Practicing the compound movements repeatedly helps you build skills and coordination through repetitive movement patterns. Training for strength helps train your neuromuscular system, thus enabling you to handle increased volume and recover faster over the long haul.

But the underlying reason for placing priority on strength first and foremost is the benefits of a solid foundation it creates for you.

Before you learn to dribble behind the back or perform a crossover in basketball, you have to learn how to dribble and keep your head up. Before you become an all-pro quarterback, you have to practice your foot mechanics and hand placement. Before you become the CEO of a top advertising agency, you have to learn the basics of marketing and consumer psychology. Before you paint a masterpiece, you have to learn how to apply the basic strokes to the canvas.

Strength in fitness isn't any different. You have to display a firm understanding and develop a general skill-set before advancing.

Mario doesn't fight Bowser at the beginning. Nor does Link fight Gannondorf at the beginning. They both level up, gathering the right tools and strength before facing their toughest foe.

Ask yourself this: Have you ever seen a jacked dude or a lean and muscular woman who didn't have a solid foundational level of strength?

No, you haven't.

You don't have to display Incredible Hulk or Juggernaut level strength, but you need a solid baseline.

This might sound terrifying to women, but even on their best strength training days, they don't produce the levels of testosterone that allow men to develop the muscles that they do. Strength helps women obtain a leaner body and a boost of confidence, and allows them to develop those shapely curves that many desire.

However, women—you're not going to build a top shelf set of glutes without lifting heavy. Men—you're not going to look like you lift without obtaining some appreciable strength.

Training for strength benefits your metabolism and trains you to be antifragile (as discussed earlier). And it's just pretty damn awesome to be strong. Being strong brings an internal sense of confidence, empowerment, independence, and badassery with it. Ladies don't need men to help with their groceries or to open the jar. Need to carry the luggage at the airport? No problem. Carry some dog food? No problem.

Training for strength allows you to use more weights once the time comes for producing more reps, hence causing greater hypertrophy (aka muscle gains). You'll recruit more muscle fibers by lifting 45 pounds after a few weeks of dedicated strength work than you will if you start week one with only 15 pounds since you didn't take the time to build your foundation.

Isolation and high-rep work comes after building your strength to a solid baseline level.

Noticing yourself becoming stronger produces a magical vibe. Each time one of my female clients completes their first unassisted pull-up, their eyes light up and they almost instantly become a new person due to accomplishing a feat that didn't seem feasible at the beginning.

When a male client deadlifts one and a half times his body weight or bench-presses his body weight, it brings about a sense of glory and pride. Once you achieve a solid baseline of strength and unlock initial goals you didn't think were possible, infinite possibilities present themselves.

All the limitations that you, society, or anyone else placed upon you vanish. Maybe you were once categorized as clumsy, weak, nonathletic, but once you accomplish some strength goals, you'll start to realize that those labels aren't permanent.

All of a sudden, through accomplishing your initial fitness goal, you'll start to have a desire to jump higher, run faster, lift heavier, and seek many other challenges. Build your foundation and the world opens up in abundant ways.

Your mission, should you choose to accept:

Challenge yourself for the next few weeks to get stronger on your main lifts for each session. Each week, try to get a little stronger (even five pounds makes a difference).

Strategy #34: Noticing the Intangibles as the First Signs of Progress

We live in a world obsessed with sex. It's all about ratcheting up the sex appeal meter. Most of our initial fitness aspirations have an underlying motivation that involves sex (it's merely human nature to want to feel desirable).

Ask any Joe or Jane walking down the street why they work out and the reason most likely entails a desire to change their appearance.

Initially, we'll hit the gym and do our due diligence in the kitchen motivated by external aspirations. We want bigger biceps. A fuller chest. Tighter arms. Tighter cores. A worthy set of glutes that prop up instead of sag down. These aspirations are fine, but as we learned in section II dealing with mindset, external motivations can only carry us so far along the motivational line. Eventually, the motivational flame driven solely by appearance and approval from others withers.

Building muscle takes time. Losing fat isn't a 100-meter sprint. It's a full marathon that requires pacing. You'll gain progress along the way, but oftentimes you'll feel as if nothing is happening. It will feel like watching paint dry.

This is why there's potential danger waiting for you around the corner.

Focusing only on how you look every day is going to stress you out and make you feel like nothing is happening due to the rate of progress. Fat loss doesn't occur linearly, so you won't necessarily have the same amount of weight slide off each week. Maybe for a week or two, your weight stagnates, while over the next few weeks, a wave of fat flies off. Fat loss is similar to human behavior—both are predictably irrational.

However, before the radical transformation occurs and new pictures of your hot body appear on social media, there's a plethora of intangibles that occur, which are the true signs of your fitness moving in a positive direction. You may desire to lose 20 pounds, but before you get close to that magic number, you need to be on the lookout for the intangibles.

What are the intangibles and why not just focus on my fat loss?

There's a fitness cliché stating, "It takes four weeks for you to notice your body changing, eight weeks for your friends to notice, and twelve weeks for the rest of the world to take notice." This is spot on in most cases. If it takes that long to notice results, then how can you sustain the momentum and encouragement needed to show up each week and work hard?

Easy, look for the intangibles. The intangibles provide positive reinforcement and confidence, and are the first indicator of your increasing skill level.

Sample questions about the intangibles to ask yourself when it comes to fat loss

"How does my body feel compared to the beginning?" "Are those achy joints not as achy?" "Is my back pain slowly disappearing due to me strengthening my glutes and hamstrings?" "Do I have more energy these days compared to pre-fitness?" "Is my appetite a little more regular (don't be afraid, this is a good sign)?"

"How's my libido?" "How's the quality of my sleep?" "How's my mobility?" "Are those tight hip flexors moving more fluidly?" "Has my mood improved over the last few weeks?" "Have I gotten stronger with my lifts?" "How's my endurance?"

The most important question to ask yourself is, "Has the quality of my life improved since I started strength training and practicing positive eating habits?"

If you answered "yes," congrats, you're on the right path. You're feeling better, moving better, and the appearance will follow suit. Think of your results in fitness progressing in sequential order as follows:

1. You get stronger

2. Your performance across all lifts increases

3. You lose fat

4. Muscles appear

Your mission, should you choose to accept:

Take a moment and ask yourself, "Has my life improved since starting a fitness habit"? If you haven't started, come back to this question two weeks after you start and be honest with yourself when assessing the impact it's having on your life (at the beginning, remember the intangibles before obsessing over appearance).

Strategy #35: Treat Your Fitness Like Your Dating Life

I have a confession to make that I use to feel embarrassed about—I'm an old-fashioned type of fella when it comes to romance.

I still believe in love. The forever kind. The type of feelings that Florentino Ariza shared for Fermina Daza in *Love in the Time of Cholera*. The type that our favorite singers have crooned and poured their hearts over throughout the years. The type we view in our favorite romantic comedies.

Ok, I'm sure you just read this and thought, "Whoa. Chill out, dude. Forever-and-ever-love? How about some coffee and then see where this goes?"

Agreed.

From the couples in those cheesy commercials explaining how online dating finally brought them true love to douchebags giving guys a bad name with their less-than-ethical approaches to the girl crying her eyes out at the cafe while I'm writing (true story), everyone is looking for love—some for one night and others for the long haul.

We all desperately want to be wanted and desired. Each day, it seems there's another online dating site sprouting up promising meaningful connections. Whether you're a yogi, a bro, a long-term seeker, a music lover, a religious person, or you name it—there's a site specifically meant for you.

Ok, I just went on a small ramble about dating and love, but what does this have to do with me becoming better with my fitness? Everything.

Why dating & fitness are inseparable

It's called the art of experimenting. Test and assess. In the dating world, it's totally normal (and highly recommended) to date until you find "the one" or at least someone who you think is "the one."

You wouldn't date someone who makes you feel crummy as a person.

You wouldn't date someone who you didn't look forward to seeing. You wouldn't date someone who makes you feel anxious and emotionally depleted after being around them. You wouldn't date someone long term who has a crazy personality (think Glen Close from *Fatal Attraction*). You wouldn't date someone who's a negative influence on your work and life.

Your fitness deserves the same amount of respect as your love life. Your love life needs attention and nurturing just as your training programs and workout environments do. You shouldn't partake in a training program that you resent. You shouldn't take on a training program that isn't sustainable just as you shouldn't date a scrub (shout-out to TLC) who doesn't bring anything to the table.

At the beginning of your fitness journey, you'll pick a routine that seems good on paper and reasonable. But you will only truly know if it's sustainable and effective for your lifestyle after trying it out. You don't know if it's true love after three dates; you won't know if it's a match made in heaven after three workouts.

We think we know what's good for us and what our type is, but often, we end up with the polar opposite. Expect and embrace this with your fitness. Heavy lifting may not be your flavor at first, but after a few dates, you start to warm up to it and love blossoms. Next thing you know, you're a strength-training enthusiast with a soft spot for power lifting. Maybe you're a self-professed loner, but the community-oriented atmosphere of CrossFit brings out a side you didn't know existed—now exercise and motivation isn't an issue.

Keep experimenting until you find a routine that fits your preferred lifestyle and meshes flawlessly with your specific physique goals. There is no perfect workout routine or training program. But there are training programs that are more optimal and better suited for specific goals than others. Don't feel ashamed or bummed out about exploring different forms of training at the beginning. At least you'll figure out what you like and don't like. This will save you wasted time and money (in more ways than one).

With full body splits (exercising your entire body with all muscles being worked in one workout), body part splits (separating your muscle groups to be worked on different days), and many more, the options to achieve your fitness goals are as abundant as the options you have in dating. Stay with an abundance mindset, never a scarcity mindset. Just as you'll date someone to see if there is chemistry that will potentially brew, date your training program to see if you two will vibe together (just give it more than one chance/workout).

Your mission, should you choose to accept:

Go on a date. Not an actual date with another human but with your fitness. Choose a type of strength training that interest you and give it a shot. Who knows, maybe sparks will fly and love will blossom in front of your eyes. After all, Lionel Richie did sing about love conquering all. On second thought, go on a date with another human as well (life is short), but get your workout in first.

Strategy #36: Avoid Shiny-Object Syndrome & Allow the Magic to Happen

Start…Start over…Start again…And start back over once again. Sound familiar? How about this.

Do you have fifteen amazing business ideas in your head and a few jotted down on your notepad, but not one actual up-and-running business? Did you buy a few online courses so you can turn a passion into a career, but you haven't made it through one module yet? Maybe you were training for an upcoming marathon, but something came up (again) that prevented you from participating in the event.

Do you use online dating sites and experience many wonderful first dates but have doubts because your latest match just may be the one? (There are just so many choices, it's hard to turn down those matches.)

Here's a biggie—you change your workout routine every two weeks because you gotta keep your muscles guessing and you'll plateau if you don't keep them confused.

While I'm not a doctor, this is a picture-perfect example of Shiny Object Syndrome (SOS).

This type of person always starts things, but never finishes them. People who suffer from SOS get distracted by new ideas and thoughts (often impulsive), whether their own or others. They lose themselves in fantasies, imaginations of what ifs, and dreaming away without actually sticking to anything and doing the necessary work.

Each day, all of us are confronted with potential SOS scenarios—emails from marketers promising to automate some boring process of our business, gurus promising to get us rich in less time with their three secrets, and fitness magicians promising to get rid of our extra weight in less time if we follow their secret formula.

This syndrome isn't fatal or impossible to recover from—you just need to become aware and not react to your impulsive thoughts. Realize that whatever you're going after or creating requires time to come to fruition (no other way around it).

Displaying patience is damn hard living in today's microwave generation. Patience has become obsolete in our society. What is hard work? What is earning something the old-fashioned way? Patience, while far from the sexiest of topics, is one of the most important attributes for success in life and fitness.

Love and fitness need time to blossom

How about this.

You find someone you like, and you stay with that person and allow your casual relationship to potentially blossom into a serious relationship.

Common sense right?

If you like someone that gels with your lifestyle and world perspectives, you should give it time to see where it leads you. Your fitness programs operate under the same umbrella. After playing the field for a bit, you settle down with the right one and don't cheat on them (that's bad karma and breaking code).

If you commit to a full-body routine, that means you're 100% with that specific program. You're not program hopping over to this new five-day body part split after seeing the latest *Muscle & Fitness* magazine. You're not going to give up on your new program after only three weeks because catastrophic results didn't manifest.

You don't marry someone after three weeks. You may like them and things might be going well, but that doesn't mean it's time to ring the bells. Maybe the person you're dating has a minor character trait that ticks you off and you get into a mini argument one night—that doesn't mean the relationship is doomed.

A flower doesn't fully blossom on day five. Luke Skywalker wasn't the baddest Jedi in the galaxy in three weeks. Jamiroquai wasn't the greatest band and full of awesomeness within two weeks of playing. I didn't achieve my fitness goals in three weeks. Remarkable feats slowly build up over time.

Once you commit to a training program, give it four to six weeks before you make any alterations. If you're constantly changing every week, how will you know what's working and what needs to be thrown out or modified? Give your program time to run its course before hopping to the next program. No one achieves remarkability with their fitness by constantly chasing the latest shiny fitness programs.

There are no shortcuts in fitness. There are plenty of good marketers in fitness who do a tremendous job of seducing you into buying their latest "hocus pocus" fitness products. Give your body time to adapt and adjust to the program before pulling the plug. Fitness is a long-term game; refrain from reacting with an instantaneous mindset.

Your mission, should you choose to accept:

Pick a program out and stay with the exact plan for four to six weeks before making any adjustments. Give it time to work its magic.

Strategy #37: Don't Let the Scale Play Mind Games with You

The mighty scale has been the source of many tears, frustrations, and curse words. There was a time when I based all my progress on the scale, which served as the judge of my success or failure. When it comes to fat loss, the majority of people look at the scale as their barometer for progress. If their numbers are down—great, this equals progress. If they weigh a couple extra pounds—not so great. This logic is counterproductive, psychologically draining, and spiritually depleting.

Awarding the scale a leading role in determining your progress is a losing game, which leads to your self-worth and confidence spiraling down the toilet. While weight loss happens along your fitness journey, your primary focus is on losing fat, not just weight (an arbitrary number). Losing fat is what turns your physique into an awe-inspiring figure; losing weight is just a numbers game, not necessarily equaling the lean and muscular figure circulating in your mind.

While embarking along this journey, it's important to note that while muscle and fat might weigh the same, muscle is denser than fat and takes up less space. This explains why you may not lose as much weight as expected, but still look vastly different in front of the mirror.

If you're starting a new weight-training regimen, you might gain a few pounds initially.

What do you mean? Keep calm and take a breath.

This is common for newer users and those coming back from a long layoff due to various hormonal factors and extra water within your cells compensating for the inflammation going on within your muscle cells.

Anytime we see a rise on the scale, we think that we've added fat onto our bodies. However, keep in mind that fat accumulates and is lost at a moderate pace. Weight fluctuating over the course of days is normal. I tend to fluctuate around five pounds myself. To keep some sanity, I recommend that you throw the scale away. (Ok, maybe not literally, since you paid money for it. But, you should at least hide it far away in your closet.)

A couple lifestyle factors causing your body to fluctuate in weight

Letting the scale serve as your court of opinion is going to dish out more headaches than potential benefits. Here are five common reasons for your fluctuations in weight.

1. The amount of food eaten and our stomach content – What you eat and how much you eat each day causes fluctuations in your daily weight. Having food leftovers in your gut will naturally cause you to weigh more. Eating steaks all day will cause you to weigh more compared to just downing protein shakes all day (gimme the steaks each time).

If you drink copious amounts of water every day, that can cause fluctuations in your body due to increased fluids. It's a good thing to stay hydrated, due to its pivotal role in your performance and daily functioning in and out of the gym.

2. Carbohydrates – Carbohydrates are stored in our liver and muscles in the form of glycogen (a storage hangout for glucose—what gives you energy).

Since carbohydrates are stored in our muscles as glycogen, that brings in three times the amount of water, which is going to add more weight (a natural and necessary action for optimal health and performance in the gym). If you go out for all-you-can eat pasta or go on a sushi binge, then expect to weigh a little more the next day. Since you know this, don't freak out since you'll know this is all extra water.

3. Micronutrients – Sodium, in particular, can cause weight gain due to its water retention effects. How much sodium causes water retention is normally determined by your regular sodium intake. If you normally consume around 1500mg, then one day consume 4000mg, prepare to feel a little bloated due to extra water hanging around.

4. Creatine – Creatine helps increase our power and strength (that's a good thing). It is also known to cause us to hold a couple extra pounds due to its preference of hanging out in our muscle cells while pulling water in with its awesome charm (I added the charm part, but the rest is true).

5. Stress and hormones – This is a lifestyle metric that influences our sleep patterns, our calories consumed, and our activity levels. If cortisol levels spike, then fat loss comes to a screeching halt along with a wave of water retention.

Cortisol levels become wacky at times due to lack of sleep, huge caloric deficits with tons of activity (cardio or excessive weight training), and our daily stressors. While stress never goes away completely, it's definitely manageable. Most of the things we stress about aren't worth it in the grand scheme of things.

3 simple ways to assess progress

1. Bring that tape out and measure – Your goal is to lose fat, while adding as much muscle as possible. With that said, the number on the scale might not change much, but your body will look different. Taking measurements biweekly is one of best methods to track your progress and remind yourself of true progress.

2. Keep up with your performance in the gym – How do you know if you're heading in the right direction when you don't track your workouts? Are you getting stronger? Are your prescribed rest periods becoming easier? Are you able to hit all your reps with ease?

The way you're performing in the gym is an excellent indication for how you're progressing. If you're feeling like doo-doo, adjust your calories, make training modifications, or investigate further into your daily lifestyle habits.

3. Smile for the camera – Taking pictures is an honest and no BS method to determine your progress. Glancing at yourself in the mirror is awesome, but are you being truthful? Are you sucking in your stomach and how can you remember what you looked like last week?

Be objective and take photos. Eliminate your biases. It might be difficult at first, due to you seeing your "perceived trouble spots" and exposing yourself. But remember, who you are today doesn't have to be the person you are in the future.

Your mission, should you choose to accept:

If you're using the scale as your measure of progress or self-worth, throw it in the closet. After doing so, pick one of the three ways from above and use that as your measure of progress and accomplishment.

Strategy #38: Don't Skip on the Cardio, but Instead Approach in a Logical Manner

"**I** want to get lean and toned...how much cardio should I do?" "I hate cardio. But that's the only way I can lose this fat." "I run three miles four times a week. I'm going to try to bump it up to five times to lose more of this fat." "I use the elliptical every day for 40 minutes...Should I increase the time to quicken my fat loss results?" "I heard [insert a thousand different things] is the best kind of cardio?" Ask ten different people about cardio and you'll get ten different answers.

A brief introduction to cardio

Cardio is the old faithful buzzword of the fitness industry. Many pointless debates across various forums and social media outlets occur because of this word (clean eating comes in a distant second). Your heart (which means cardio) and blood vessels (which means vascular) are the two main components of your cardiovascular system.

The biggest benefit cardio provides is turning our bodies into a stronger and more efficient system. Our heart, for example, is a muscle, therefore training makes it stronger and allows more capillaries to deliver more oxygen into our muscle cells. This leads our cells to burn more fat.

Ok, we got the physiological portion out of the way.

Most people view cardio as long and slow distance activities such as biking, hiking, and going for long runs. However, cardio includes other activities such as strength training, your favorite boot camps, spin classes, body pump classes, CrossFit, swimming, salsa dancing, jump roping, and getting busy between the sheets.

If it raises your heart rate while subsequently causing heavier breathing (or panting)—that's cardio.

With that knowledge in mind, this leads to another question...

Is there a wrong type of cardio? No.

Is there a wrong type of cardio for fat loss? Yes.

Here's a better question.

Are there specific types of cardio that are more optimal depending on your goal? Absolutely.

The three main types of cardio

Most people's goal for performing cardio is fat loss, so we'll keep that in mind as we approach these three types below.

1. Low-intensity cardio – At this intensity, your heart rate will hover around 40-50% of maximum. This relaxing and simple form of cardio is excellent for beginners and valuable for advanced trainees as well. It's often performed for longer amounts of time. A prime example of low-intensity cardio is walking (underrated and boring to most, but sneakily effective).

My preferred way to implement low-intensity cardio is to stick it in (no pun intended) after your strength training session, first thing in the morning for 20–40min, or as an excuse to go out for a late evening stroll.

2. Moderate/Medium-intensity training – When the majority of people think of cardio, this type of training comes to mind. This type of training is endurance training—jogging and running on the treadmill or outside. Another word for this is steady state cardio. This type of training occurs at 60–75% of your maximum heart rate and sessions last between 30–45 minutes, excluding marathons (obviously).

Would I recommend this type of training? On most occasions, I wouldn't.

I mostly advise and coach clients that are limited with their time while being interested in improving their general health, transforming their physique, and reaching performance goals. Unless they are training for endurance events, then this type of cardio doesn't yield high enough rewards for a fat-loss nor muscle-gaining program (especially when people are already limited with their time).

How many lean and muscular individuals are hopping on the elliptical or running on the treadmill each day as their main tool for transforming their physique?

Zero.

Running on treadmills or using other cardio machines isn't wrong or committing a fitness sin, it's just not placing you in the best and most effective position to succeed with your goals. If your ideal physique involves an athletic look with appreciable amounts of muscle and definition, weight training is priority number one while cardio gets in where it fits in.

The main issue with excessive cardio

Besides wasting more time than needed, long steady state cardio can wreak havoc on our bodies, causing cortisol levels to spike. Cortisol (your stress hormone), when high, is more likely to store body fat (often in our midsections) since it's sensing your body is under appreciable amounts of stress (e.g., long runs, excessive strength training, less than stellar sleep habits, or life in general).

Excessive cardio leads to increased hunger, which is a precursor to binge eating and cyclic food behaviors. This increase in food intake is often in the form of carbohydrates (most often junk food).

There are more effective and efficient alternatives to long-distance running. Examples include strength training, jumping rope, rowing, sprinting, pushing sleds, circuit training, basketball, sand volleyball, CrossFit, and kettlebell swings.

Doesn't running on the treadmill and elliptical burn lots of calories?

Yes. However, the big picture isn't being told. Any type of training burns calories, but training isn't our main weapon for fat loss. Our nutrition is our main weapon. Our training is for strengthening and constructing a lean, high performing, and muscular physique. When you hop on the treadmill or elliptical and set your timer for 35 minutes, you'll burn plenty of calories. However, you can have sex as well and burn calories.

Here's the biggie.

After you hop off those machines, the calorie burning stops. With weight training, the calorie burning continues after the session has ended. Thus, lifting weights burns more calories overall compared to running. In the grand scheme of things, cardio (medium steady state aerobic training) isn't a necessity for fat loss.

In a highly popular research study reported in the *International Journal of Sports Nutrition*, researchers tracked 91 women who performed moderate aerobic exercise for 45 minutes, five days a week. At the conclusion of the twelve weeks, this group of women experienced little to no effect on their body composition (i.e., little fat loss) compared to a similar group who focused on diet alone.

I can't say it enough—fat loss is through diet, not your cardio. Strength training shapes your body (i.e., body composition) while placing a priority on cardio delivers the opposite.

In a study published in *The Journal of the American College of Nutrition*, there was an aerobic group who exercised four times weekly while a resistance-training group exercised three times weekly. Both groups experienced an increase in their VO2 max. VO2 max is a measure of the maximum volume of oxygen that you can use. This maximum oxygen consumption establishes your aerobic physical peak (i.e., it determines just how good of shape you're in).

Back to the research study: the strength-training group lost more fat, didn't lose lean body mass, and improved their metabolism. On the other hand, the aerobic group lost lean body mass, decreased their metabolism, and didn't improve their body composition.

3. High-intensity cardio (HIIT) – This type of training is usually done around 80-100% of your heart rate for short amounts of time. Exercises such as hill sprints, kettlebell swings, battle ropes, barbell or dumbbell complexes (i.e., a series of exercises executed in succession with the same weight), strength circuits, or sled work fit the bill. Another benefit with this type of cardio is that it helps lead to lean muscle gains besides having amazing sweat sessions.

In recent years, research has sprouted up touting the benefits of high-intensity training and how overrated long-distance training (i.e., aerobic training) is for fat loss.

Here's a review by Stephen Boutcher who states, "Most exercise protocols designed to induce fat loss have focused on regular steady state exercise such as walking and jogging at a moderate intensity. Disappointingly, these kinds of protocols have led to negligible weight loss." In that same 2008 study published in the journal *Obesity* by Boutcher and others:

"Women who performed 20 minutes of interval training for only three days a week experienced significant differences in total body fat compared to the women who performed 40 minutes of steady cardio."

What this means and a key summary to keep in mind for your cardio approach

- Focus on your diet, training plan, lifestyle, and stress management for fat loss before incorporating multiple cardio sessions.

- If you're just starting out with a training plan, go easy on the cardio and use it only when you've started to hit a wall (i.e., plateau).

- Feel free to perform one to three high intensity sessions a week once well adjusted to your lifting program, but don't overdo it—you still need time for rest and recovery.

- Approach cardio from a steady and relaxing mindset (think walking) or high intense (HIIT) mindset. Avoid the middle ground.

- If you must find outside activity to do besides strength training or going for runs, walk, dance, or have sex for extra calorie burn and mental release (writers block, stress, and everything in between will be cured).

- If your ideal physique is that of a sprinter, football player, some hot person you saw at the beach, some girl at the gym, or a tight, lean, and toned body, then throw running to the curb for now and make strength training your main focus.

- If you're an avid distance runner or take part in triathlons, then keep running (this is your life after all).

- Love endurance training, but still want to lose some fat? Then swap some of your long runs with some moderate ones and still strength train two to three days a week.

- Keep running if that's your form of medication or your way to find your inner peace. Just don't overdo it and pay attention to how your body feels.

Your mission, should you choose to accept:

Decide what your ideal physique entails. Once you've decided, choose your cardio approach to mirror the ideal physique you're pursuing. However, before implementing a cardio program, make sure your diet, training, and lifestyle is under control before adding another stressor. Start by adding one session weekly, then increase as progress stalls and comfort increases within the program.

Strategy #39: Walking Isn't Sexy, but Is Still Valuable, Therapeutic, & Nothing to Scoff At

"Walking is man's best medicine."

—Hippocrates

Let's say you're a sedentary adult and strength training isn't your cup of tea or you're just not ready for that type of commitment. Cool. Eventually you'll come around to it. In the meantime, you still want to improve your health biomarkers and lose some weight.

What shall you do?

Simple. Put a comfortable pair of shoes on and get to walking. Increase your daily step count. In all honesty, if you clean up your diet and increase your daily activity levels through walking, that will be plenty to kick-start your weight loss.

Walking isn't going to get you shredded nor dramatically enhance your physique in any form or fashion. But, it's a damn good start for someone who isn't mentally ready to start strength training and hasn't performed any type of exercise in years but wants to improve their general health.

Walking is meditative, therapeutic, improves your general health biomarkers, and serves as an excellent tool to burn extra calories without interfering with your recovery process from training.

What are some benefits to walking?

Some might call it daydreaming, others will claim it's a "trance state," and if you want to impress, you can call it "reverie." The point is, the benefits of walking extend beyond boosting your mood and uncluttering your mind from garbage—it sparks your creativity to new heights. Walking opens your world up, frees your imagination, and leaves the narrowness of your thoughts behind.

It's no wonder so many great writers and philosophers such as Charles Darwin, Jack Kerouac, Robert Louis Stevenson, Immanuel Kant, Frederiche Nietzche, William Wordsworth, and Jean-Jacques Rousseau were devoted walkers.

Various health sources claim that 10,000 steps is a healthy daily goal. It's estimated that 1000 steps are accomplished in about 10 minutes. Doing some basic math, this equals an hour of daily walking, which isn't too bad, especially for the city folks out there. Take the stairs, park further away, walk at lunch and after work to hit your quota.

Besides requiring zero equipment, having a low risk of injury, and serving as a way to easily increase the quality of your life, walking has a slew of other benefits, such as...

- Benefits toward fat loss (a little) – Walking won't turn you into superhero shape, but it will initiate the process toward becoming a superhero

- Increased longevity (or at least the quality of your life)

- Helps with joint pain

- It levels up your brain in a multitude of ways

- It's a great stress reducer

- Helpful for your immune system

- Makes you smarter

- Great for meetings (who wants to sit in a boardroom)

- Great for dates (who wants to waste money on someone when you're not sure if they're worthy of your time or money. If they complain, you automatically know it's a no-go with this person)

- It helps keep your butt active (literally) – We live in a culture where we sit down most of the day. At work, we sit down and look at a screen all day. We head home, sit on a comfortable couch, and maybe play some video games or watch sports while we're at it. We're probably on our feet for an hour or two daily out of the sixteen to nineteen hours we're awake

- Helps with blood pressure and glucose control – Thirty minutes of walking after a meal has been shown to help decrease your blood pressure and triglyceride levels, according to the American Diabetes Association

Your mission, should you choose to accept:

Go for a daily walk, take the stairs, walk instead of driving everywhere, stand instead of opting to sit, conduct your meetings while walking, and take your date for a walk instead of the outdated movie date. Just get some extra movement into your daily life. Start small by getting an extra 20–30 minutes and increase from there.

Strategy #40: Get Some Hobbies, Enjoy Life, & Place a Priority on Your Rest & Recovery

We'll work our butts off in the weight room, sweat will drench our faces, and we'll strain for that last rep. Yet, while we're juggernauts in the weight room, we turn a blind eye to our recovery methods.

I get it.

Rest and recovery aren't nearly as sexy as squats, hip thrusts, deadlifts, fanciful food pictures, and sexy perfectly angled bodies.

Ever wondered why you see those regulars in the gym who haven't made significant progress in years, even though they consistently weight train, perform cardio, post fitness updates, and share food pictures? Nine out of ten times, it's their lack of attention toward rest and recovery that is the disconnect between their current physique and the one they aspire to.

Proper rest and recovery is the missing link.

You can have the greatest workouts in the world and an optimal diet plan, but without the proper amount of rest, you're going to progress at a snail's pace (and that's being generous).

Why you need to rest

Let's go on a brief journey.

You walk into the gym and perform an intense strength training session. As you're lifting, you're breaking down muscle tissue, creating tiny tears in your muscle fibers. This is why you can't lift the same amount at the end as you could at the beginning. You're weaker and you're body is broken down (this is normal; you worked hard, after all). Now it's time to leave the gym, and this is where the magic happens. Your body begins repairing muscle tissue so you can return stronger for the next session.

Your nervous system needs rest

Each time you squat, deadlift, hip thrust, or run hill sprints, you're putting stress on your central nervous system (CNS). The more intense your workout, the greater the number of sets, the more fatigued your CNS becomes.

This is a huge reason why I'm not a fan of beginners doing body part splits (one muscle per day lifting five to six days a week at the beginning) or people doing six straight WOD's (workouts of the day), even though I still think CrossFit is good when programmed properly.

Beginners can't handle as much volume as a seasoned lifter. It's no coincidence that newbies are sore for a couple days after their first few sessions. For those who like to lift frequently at the gym, keep your daily volume under control and keep sessions around 35–60 minutes.

Prevent injuries by paying attention to feedback from your body

Do you have that ache in your knees each time you squat or lunge? Is your achy shoulder, tennis elbow, golf elbow, or back pain giving you problems each time you touch a weight?

Providing you're exercising with sound technique, you're likely not giving your body enough time to heal and loading too much too soon. While muscles can grow at a decent rate, our joints and smaller tissues take a little longer to adapt to your ever-increasing strength. Loading too much, too soon, can lead to nagging pains.

Not paying attention to these little pains in your shoulder, that nagging shin pain on every squat, or the ankle pain whenever you run eventually leads to something bigger that can put you on the shelf for months.

Relax, you still need to live life

It's easy to become obsessed with being fit and healthy, leaving other areas of life out of the picture. This isn't sustainable or fun in the long term. Who wants to sacrifice hanging out with friends or whatever other hobbies you have in order to become fit and lean?

Doesn't sound worth it in my book. Looking awesome and feeling good doesn't mean losing touch with friends and your identity. Developing a one-track mind leads to a skewed attitude toward food and exercise over the long haul. Instead of devoting yourself to the gym and working out 24/7, here are some alternatives to occupy you while you rest and allow your body to heal.

- Sleep (quiet the room, keep it dark, and aim for a minimum of seven hours)
- Immerse yourself in a great book
- Listen to music that moves your soul
- Go on a stimulating date
- Go for a mind-clearing walk
- Take a yoga class
- Meditate for as little as five minutes
- Foam roll & get to know the lacrosse ball (your body will send plenty of thanks)
- Get a massage
- Have an unapologetic dance party (solo ones are just as effective)
- Try a salsa dance class (like me) or any other type of dance class
- Hydrate and eat well

Your mission, should you choose to accept:

Instead of focusing on doing more and more, I challenge you to try a new hobby or activity this week. Stretching ourselves outside our comfort zones isn't a bad thing; once you stop learning and expanding, you stop growing. Try new hobbies and learn new subjects, and you're one step closer to becoming a Renaissance man or woman.

Section VI

Bonus Strategies

I'm a huge fan of superhero movies and one of the best moments during the movie experience is the anticipation of the end credit scene.

Keeping this in mind, I attempted my version of the end credits scene. Or to use concert lingo—the encore. The encore doesn't need extra explanation; the audience just wants to hear you jam away for a few more songs.

The end credits scene doesn't need to be long; the audience just wants to leave on a good note, feeling excited about what they just witnessed and what's to come.

This bonus section has important points, and each of these bonus topics enhances the quality of your fitness life while simultaneously boosting your personal life. Without further ado, here are the final points to conclude your journey to constructing a world-class body and living the good life.

Bonus strategy #1: Everything is a Stressor

Stress is a popular topic. We hear about it in news reports (often bad news), in books promising to unlock the secrets to managing stress, and from gurus on television who guarantee to make stress pull a disappearing act. Most of the time, stress is portrayed as the villain due to the negative effect it has on our bodies. While stress can hamper our fat loss, we wouldn't be alive without a little bit of stress.

A brief reminder about the positives of stress

Stress plays a pivotal role in our flight-or-fight system, helping guide us in potentially dangerous and high-pressure situations. Besides these events, a little bit of stress (in moderation of course) has been shown to help our...

- **Cognitive function** – A 2013 study by the University of California, Berkeley, concluded that moderate amounts of stress can lead to cell growth in the brain's learning centers.

  Other benefits include sharpening our focus. Think about having to make life-or-death decisions in the wild. You don't want to be thinking about how pretty the tree is beside you when a predator is staring you down. Another situation is focusing and recalling information during exams and important meetings. In those times, thinking about the dinner you had last night isn't going to serve you.

- **Longevity** – Researchers at the University of Wisconsin-Madison surveyed close to 29,000 people to rate their stress levels over the past year and how much it influenced their health. The choices were a little, a moderate amount, or a lot.

Over the next eight years, public death records were used to record the passing of anyone in this study. The conclusions were that those who perceived high levels of stress and believed it to have large impact on their health had a 43% increased chance of dying. Those who experienced plenty of stress but didn't perceive it as a negative were the least likely group of all to die.

What does this mean?

Mostly, that your thoughts and perceptions are powerful forces. You choose to believe what you think and feel (remember the belief section earlier in the book). Change your perception; your reality will change.

- **Increased performance** – Besides your brain receiving a boost, your endurance and physical performance across various metrics will increase.

Why is this?

In heightened situations, whether it's running from tigers or running a marathon, your body will release a hormone called adrenaline, which increases your heart rate, thus speeding up your metabolism. Adrenaline helps you fight fatigue, tiredness, or pain while increasing your reactions and reflexes.

Stress isn't all bad. But it's still a thorn in many people's sides when it comes to their daily life and eventually letting those issues affect their fitness lives.

Managing stress within our fitness and daily lives

Everything is a stressor, thus completely removing it from your life is not going to happen. While you can't eliminate all stressors from your life, you can reframe how you view those stressors. The obvious sources of stress involve work, home life, friends nagging us, spouses, financial situations, worrying about the future, and worrying about other random uncertainties going on within our lives.

Did you realize that training, running, and any other physical activity is a stressor as well?

It's true. Strength training causes stress within our system. This isn't bad per se, because our bodies need some stress.

Why did I preach about sleep and cortisol earlier when all stress isn't bad?

As with everything in life, too much of anything has its drawbacks. Training and stress are no exceptions. Too much stress will raise your cortisol to unhealthy levels. This subsequently slows your fat loss.

I've dealt with clients, oftentimes busy professionals, creatives, entrepreneurs, and various high achievers, who weren't losing fat even though they were training regularly and watching what they ate.

What was the deal?

Their daily volume of stress. Not enough attention was given to the overall structure of their lives. Each of these individuals had very demanding lifestyles with work and personal responsibilities, or was currently involved during a hectic period of work and didn't account for that.

Whether you're an accountant and it's tax season, a creative professional working on a demanding project for your client, a medical orthopedic resident working 10+ hour days, or an entrepreneur hustling daily to raise his business off the ground, you must factor in the stress from your work and personal life and adjust your training.

The more stress in your life, the more demanding hours you have at work, the less demanding your training program and frequency needs to be. This isn't an excuse not to work hard during your workouts. This means that instead of opting for your normal five-day routine, you drop down to a more manageable three-day full-body routine to compensate for your demanding work schedule while still giving yourself plenty of time for rest and recovery.

At the end of the day, no matter how hard and intense you train, you need to sleep and rest on a consistent basis. Sleeping more trumps opting for an extra workout (no ifs, ands, or buts). An easy way to manage this pendulum of work and training is to forecast ahead.

If you know that the current quarter is your busy season or that this particular month in the hospital is demanding or that you have an important business proposal due, drop into a maintenance training plan where your only goal is to complete the minimum in order to keep what you got and not slip up.

However, when work slows down and life isn't abnormally hectic, increase the intensity of your workout program again.

Managing fitness and life in cohesion boils down to having periods of intense training and then periods where it's more on cruise control. Even athletes have an off-season. Periodize your training for the high and low periods based on the schedules of your work and personal life.

Your mission, should you choose to accept:

Identify some upcoming busy periods in your life; forecast ahead what you'll do with your training.

Bonus strategy #2: Embrace the Slow Burn

My patience meter was nonexistent at one point in time. I wanted big biceps rivaling Popeye, sculpted shoulders carved out of stone, and most important, I wanted the appearance of a powerful and mighty superhero.

It's good to have goals and ambitions, but I shouldn't have expected these results after only seven workouts. Oftentimes, our patience betrays us and becomes our worst enemy.

In effort to prevent our patience from turning to the dark side of the fitness force, let's go back to grade school and learn from the tortoise and the hare. *The Tortoise and the Hare* is a timeless classic that displays how patience can become your best ally. The tortoise displayed that taking action methodically and making progress in a slow and steady manner trumps the fast-acting habits of the hare. The majority of situations in life benefit those with methodical and precise approaches and a slow and steady mindset.

By adopting the slow burn, as I call it, you won't flame out or wither away after a minute (that's never a good thing, if you catch my drift). The slow burn method is attainable and sustainable. Just as companies don't instantly become billion-dollar empires, fat loss isn't going to happen instantly. Expecting these kinds of results will leave you disappointed and resentful, which will most likely lead you to quit fitness in a couple of weeks. As you go along your journey and adopt the slow burn approach, keep these four reminders in your brain at all times.

1. Focus on your why, not how or when – You might feel dazed and confused at times, uncertain about your skills, but that means nothing as long as you remember your purpose for embarking along your specific fitness journey.

2. Keep an open mind – Slow and steady is only a problem when you're miserable throughout the process, so find a method that you 100% vibe with. Enjoy the journey and the process of growing into a better you.

3. Pay no attention to the voices of self-doubt and stay away from haters – Some people don't want to see you succeed because then they'll have no excuse for not getting their asses off the couch and striving for greatness. Your goals and successes are far more important than some random Joe or Jane's opinion.

4. Keep your vehicle in the correct lane – If any situation or decision isn't in alignment with your purpose in fitness and life—don't do it. You'll see gimmicky fitness products promising rapid weight loss in four weeks. If it sounds too good to be true, it probably is.

The more connected and aligned you are with your vision, the easier it'll be to show up each day. Sometimes the reason why you aren't succeeding with a particular goal isn't because of effort, but instead, because that goal isn't in alignment with who you are.

Your mission, should you choose to accept:

Assess your current fitness situation. Are you putting unnecessary pressure on yourself to achieve your goals? Are they unrealistic? If so, slow down and set some reasonable goals. Set these goals in a way that allows you to enjoy your daily life while reaching your fitness goals.

Bonus strategy #3: Those Glutes Don't Lie: Make Glute Training a Priority

We're officially living in the age of the glutes. Gone are the days of obsessing over abs and arms and in its place is an obsession over glutes. Nothing is more trendy and in demand than a nice pair of glutes. This isn't just about women obtaining a nice set of glutes; it's for us men as well. Beach muscles are cool, but that was so 2011.

Ladies, if you aren't hitting the glutes heavily and frequently, it's time to change the routine. Guys, if you aren't hitting the glutes heavily and frequently, now's the time—lay off the bench press, bicep curls, and tricep kickbacks.

This glute movement isn't just about aesthetics and looking fantastic at the beach. Our glutes serve a prominent role in our body and affect our performance in the gym.

The glutes are the largest set of muscles in the human body and the strongest. Therefore, working this group of muscles will cause a greater metabolic effect within the body (i.e., burn more calories). Your glutes will increase your strength in practically every lift. That back pain that you complain about that sometimes debilitates you is caused by weak glutes; other areas of your body must compensate for droopy glutes.

A strong set of glutes improves your posture, helps stabilize your hips, and will help fight against father time by preventing a saggy butt. If you're into athletics, your glutes play a pivotal role in your speed and various explosive movements (there's a reason why track and field athletes have some of the best bodies on this planet).

I could talk all day about the glutes, but let's keep this party moving along.

A brief primer on how to train your glutes

Glutes need to be trained frequently and for varying rep ranges to elicit maximum growth. We use our glutes plentifully each day just like our calves, so they can handle high volume. In the training programs that I write out for clients who want to take their glutes to the next level, they work the glutes almost every training session. It's not necessary to do a ton of sets; it's the frequency, execution of the lift, and variations of rep ranges that creates the magic (i.e., jeans filling out, turning heads at the grocery store, etc.).

Separate your glute training into these three ranges when designing your glute work:

1. Heavy work – This is generally lower rep work ranging from three to seven reps. As we mentioned earlier, strength is highly important and serves as our training foundation.

2. Middle tier range work – This will be around eight to fifteen reps. This is probably the most common rep range for fitness enthusiast and is also known as the hypertrophy range. The time under tension is a little longer here, thus eliciting a little more muscle recruitment compared to the lower rep work, which is more neurologically based.

3. High rep work – This work range is all about getting the butt burns (yes, your butt will literally feel like it's on fire). This is mostly endurance and burnout work. Normally, these kinds of sets are perfect to end your workout with. Some of the best equipment to use for these sets is bands and bodyweight movements. Rep ranges are normally from 16–30 reps.

As you structure your glute training, your heavy strength work is at the very beginning and then as you progress through the workout, you can start to implement the higher rep work since the percentage of weight you're using isn't as close to your max as the strength work was. As you're designing a glute workout and incorporating these into your regimen, here are a couple of my favorite glute exercises.

- BB Hip thrust (my favorite, the granddaddy of them all)
- BB glute bridges
- Band hip thrust
- Deadlifts (sumo, jefferson, snatch grip, and conventional)
- BB squats
- BB or Db Romanian deadlifts
- Db hyperextensions
- Db or BB High step ups
- Bulgarian split squats
- Bodyweight single leg hip thrust
- Bodyweight hip thrust
- Hill sprints (for my cardio lovers)

Your mission, should you choose to accept:

If you're not working your glutes, start during your next workout. Implement one or two of these movements into each of your workouts. Some might feel initially uncomfortable, but with practice, you'll make perfect. Remember, glutes raise your sex appeal tenfold.

Bonus strategy #4: How to Make Your Workouts Shorter, but Just As (if not more) Efficient

We're busy people trying to make our unique dent in the universe, have adventures, take in experiences, take care of families (some of us), and live the good life. The gym is a tiny fraction of the life equation for the majority of us (me included).

We don't have time for multiple 90-minute workouts throughout the week (nor is this even necessary). At times, some of us don't have the time to even get multiple 45-minute workouts in—which is totally understandable.

We all have those abnormally hectic weeks. Luckily, there are a plethora of methods that can reduce our time in the gym, while still providing us with one hell of a workout. There's no need to camp out at the gym and participate in marathon sessions when you have other important events to attend.

You don't have to train your muscles to failure, lift till you feel like puking, and train balls to wall. All you need to do is train sensibly and approach your fitness from an intelligent standpoint—know what your goals are, how much time you have, and how demanding the other stressors in your life currently are.

With that said, here are a couple methods I use when on the road, when I need to shorten my sessions while maintaining proper intensity, or when I need a good change of pace.

1. Supersets – This is the easiest method to use. The majority of my workouts are structured in this format by default. Supersets are simply performing one exercise right after another one. You can jump immediately into the next exercise or you can take a brief time in between each one.

The rest periods between exercises are dependent upon your training level. Most of the time, I have clients take 30–45 seconds in between each exercise since I still want them to recover a little in order to have some appreciable strength on the subsequent exercise. The only time I jump back and forth is when it's a weighted exercise proceeded by a bodyweight or plyometric activity.

Ex: 1a) BB deadlifts superset with 1b) db bench press. Take 30–45 seconds rest in between

Or

EX: 1a) BB squats superset with 1b) Bodyweight jump squats. Proceed immediately to 1b after 1a

2. Density training – Ever since reading Charles Staley's *Muscle Logic: Escalating Density Training* years ago, this has become my favorite training method. I'm able to combine conditioning and strength work. A basic premise for this style of training is to set a prescribed amount of time, for example, fifteen minutes, and go back and forth through your exercises until the time is up.

The basic method is to pick two or three exercises that don't compete against each other and take around 30 seconds in between each for the entire 15 minutes. This method is flexible for a muscle-gaining program as well as a badass method for fat loss. If you care about strength, no problem; keep the reps lower during the allocated time. More concerned about fat loss? Bump the reps up to the middle tier range.

Your mission, should you choose to accept:

Next time you're pressed for time, incorporate one of these training methods into your workout instead of not working out at all.

Bonus strategy #5: Lessons from Allen Iverson & Adding Some "Funtronics" to Your Life & Fitness

At end of the day, we're not performing brain surgery, building a space shuttle, scheming on how to reach Saturn, debating over world peace, or delivering a defense case in the court of law.

We're only exercising. Or as my favorite basketball player of all time, Allen Iverson, states, "We talkin' about practice...Practice man...Practice, not the game, but practice."

We talkin' about fitness...not surgery...not the stock market...not world peace...not quantum physics...But fitness.

It's only squats, push-ups, and some jump roping. At the end of the day, whether you're into CrossFit, bodybuilding, Olympic lifting, athletics, or power lifting, it doesn't matter. We're all just trying to be our ultimate selves, look good naked, and have some adventures while living the good life. If you find yourself tempted to defend yourself in a fitness pissing contest (over the Internet or the water cooler), I beg you not to succumb. Instead, I want you to remember, "We talkin' about fitness."

You have better things to do with your life than argue about the optimal ratio of protein per meal or the optimal angle for maximum recruitment of the biceps or the exact moment we should ingest our BCAA's before and after our workouts. No one really cares who lifts more. No one notices if your left pec is a couple inches smaller than your right. I promise, no one cares about your style of training or what your max is on the bench press.

Just eat tasty and satiating food. Get your sweat on. Lift some heavy weights. Make sleep a "no ifs, ands, or buts" activity. Treat people well. Go out and dance. Maybe get lucky and turn that long distance crush into a reality. Be remarkable. Make your unique dent in the universe whichever way you deem appropriate.

One of my good friends, when asked what he majored in, used to reply with the major "funtronics."

If it isn't fun or pleasurable and instead is causing regret and negative feelings, kick it to the curb and try something else. Add some "funtronics" to your fitness and live the good life.

Your mission, should you choose to accept:

This is the easiest one...Add some "funtronics" to your life (however you deem appropriate).

Section VII

Outro

Epilogue: Are You Ready to Walk the Path?

"It's your road, and yours alone. Others may walk it with you, but no one can walk it for you."

—Rumi

A Japanese proverb states, *"Vision without action is a daydream. Action without vision is a nightmare."*

When it comes to succeeding in fitness, we must let our vision guide us and serve as our compass, while letting our actions propel us to new heights (i.e., building a world-class body while living a world-class lifestyle).

Easy peasy right?

Not so much. The idea of fitness is pretty damn easy and straightforward on paper, but once you start throwing in all the other facets of our lives, succeeding in fitness isn't a slam dunk. Bad situations, inconveniences, and unexpected circumstances are going to intervene and interfere with our fitness goals.

We can choose to indulge in self-pity, become robots in our daily lives, and give up, or we can choose to accept the circumstances and fight for what we desire. For a period of time, I forgot that I had a choice.

This book was conceived during a dark period for me. I wasn't working out. My eating habits were suffering. My behaviors were sporadic and I was treating the people around me horribly. My depression was taking over while my anxiety was at an all-time high. I was all over the place. I wanted to change. I wished for my old body. My fitness identity vanished.

The only way I could change, reinvent myself, and get my fitness life back in order was to return to square one—the basics. Without a solid foundation emphasizing the proper mindset and installing positive habits, your training program and diet mean little. The basics come before anything. The basics create the framework needed for lasting success.

Before you can learn fancy salsa patterns, you have to learn your basic step count and develop your footwork. Before an NBA player is an all-star, he has to learn how to dribble. A world-class pitcher isn't possible without proper throwing mechanics.

As we learned earlier, developing belief and confidence in yourself like Marvin Gaye is essential to surviving an uncertain and unpredictable journey. You have to practice, show up each day, and clock your 10,000 hours like Jackson Pollack, Michael Jordan, and many other talented artists and athletes.

No matter your current situation, no matter how many times you've tried before, and no matter the opinions of others, there's always time to change your projected fitness story arc. Most important, there's time to change your projected story arc when it comes to living a rich and fulfilled life.

Throughout the book, this path has been forged. You've been warned about what potentially lies ahead. You know it won't be easy. You know you're more than enough, despite what anyone else might have to say. You know the model that's needed for success with your mindset, nutrition, training, and desired lifestyle.

However, even with all this information presented, there's a monumental decision ahead for you. It's a decision that you and only you can make.

Will you actually follow through with the desire you have for better health, more confidence, a richer life, and a leaner physique?

I'm delighted and honored that you read this book and have made it this far, but this is only a small fraction of the equation. You've discovered your "why." You know how starting and succeeding with fitness can create ripples within your life. You have the proper vision established. You have more than enough knowledge to start.

But will you actually do it? Or will you say tomorrow, next week, when you get more time, when you feel motivated, or whatever other excuse sprouts up?

As Morpheus tells Neo, *"There's a difference between knowing the path and walking the path."*

There's a difference between knowing you should go to the gym three to four times a week and actually doing it. There's a difference between knowing healthy foods and actually eating them. There's a difference between knowing positive habits needed for a healthy and fit life and actually doing them.

Just knowing information and what to do isn't enough—it's only the first step. You have to follow up this knowledge with action. Don't be the guy who has all the knowledge in the world but doesn't do anything with it. You can know the path and know that you should embark on this path, but your actions are going to speak the truth and expose your true character.

Walking the path is where version 2.0 forms. Walking the path is what separates the doers from the pretenders. Walking the path is damn hard at times, but the benefits and rewards are unimaginable. Walking the path instills a "somehow, someway" attitude of inevitable success. It won't be pretty, but before beauty is formed, the ugly and dark days must be endured. There are no shortcuts. Progress isn't linear. Playing the comparison game is futile and a waste of mental bandwidth.

As you embark along the path, reframe your thoughts to only positive energy, instead of worrying about failure, the opinions of others, and any other draining source of thought.

Instead of "What if I fail," ask yourself, "What if I do nothing?" or "What if I succeed?"

If you're not applying your daily energy toward your goals, dreams, health, physique, and loved ones, your energy is instead going to the opposite.

Your energy is like an elevator; it's either going up or it's going down—there isn't a sideways. Will you waste time and precious energy going down the elevator or will you use your valuable energy to lift yourself up and rise to the top of the building. We're all riding an elevator—some of us just choose to stay on the first floor instead of riding up to the penthouse suite.

Join the Community & Fail-Proof Your Fat Loss

Thanks for checking out this book. I hope the strategies shared have proven beneficial as you embark along your new fitness journey or as you attempt to restart a fitness habit. If you made it this far into the book, I feel that something within this book resonated with you.

As a way of saying thank you for choosing this book out of the many floating around, I'm offering my free five-day fat loss eCourse titled *Fail-Proof Fat Loss*. A fitness journey is far from being easy, but this doesn't mean fitness needs to be filled with confusion and resentment for choosing a healthy lifestyle.

In *Fail-Proof Fat Loss*, you'll discover the essential techniques that will guarantee success in your fat loss goals without having your daily lifestyle thrown upside down. You will learn how to lose fat in a sustainable and intelligent way, thus preventing the chances of rebound weight gain. If you're ready to walk the path and kick-start your fat loss, then join the community at <u>theartoffitnessandlife.com</u>

One Small Ask to Help My Mission

Once again, I wanted to say thank you one final time for reading this book. Out of the millions of books in existence, this book made its way into your hands and you chose to read it.

Now I'd like to ask a small favor from you. Could you please take one minute and leave a review of this book on Amazon? Complete honesty and transparency only (whether good or bad). Taking one minute out of your day to write a review makes a big difference to me personally and to my growth as a writer, and it helps me reach my goal of helping one million people. Reviews also help improve a book's Amazon rankings. Most important, these reviews increase the likelihood that future readers who find this work will know that this book is different from the rest of the "fairy-dust," "guru-loaded," "lose fat quick" schemes that circulate in the health and fitness spaces.

Until we cross paths again for our next adventure, take care, and stay prosperous my friend.

Stay awesome,

Julian

Acknowledgements

Personally and professionally, I'm grateful for the many wonderful friendships and relationships developed throughout my life. My support network has proven invaluable during the process of creating this book. As with most things in life, very little can be accomplished without the assistance of others. This book wouldn't have happened without the vast assortment of characters that are intertwined into my daily life.

I wish to personally thank the following people for their contributions to my inspiration and knowledge and other help in creating this book:

Mom, Dad, David, Josh M., Destiney, Aunt Cathy, JC, Kenton, Ashley F., Cindy A., Canaan, Leah, Claudia, Bryan T., Joseph B., Terrance P., Zaina, Jeff L., Jonathan N., Jordan H., Jonathan M., Young Choe, Michael S., Torri, Merri, Cortney, Belinda, Jessica K., Alex M., Travis H., Malcolm, Anant + many, many more…

About the Author

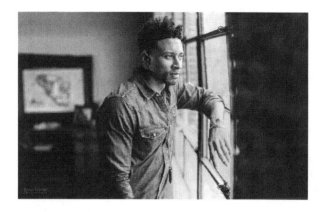

Julian Hayes II is an author, fitness and lifestyle consultant, and speaker. He founded The Art of Fitness & Life to help ambitious, creative, nerdy, and remarkable men and women build a world-class body while living a world-class lifestyle. His work has been featured in *Bodybuilding.com*, *The Huffington Post*, *MindBodyGreen*, and many more.

He loves helping men and women integrate their optimal lifestyle into a sustainable fitness habit, without having to use tricks or lose their identity through the process. He believes an optimal lifestyle and living the good life consists of fitness keeping you young, music moving your soul, books feeding your brain, and creativity driving you every day.

Made in the USA
Columbia, SC
20 February 2018